TACKLING THE SURGICAL MAZE
AN INTRODUCTION TO CLINICAL METHODOLOGY

TACKLING THE SURGICAL MAZE

AN INTRODUCTION TO CLINICAL METHODOLOGY

ARTHUR FELICE

Published by Agenda

Agenda, Miller House, Tarxien Road, Airport Way, Luqa, Malta.
Tel: (+356) 21664488 E-mail: info@millermalta.com

Produced by Perfecta Advertising Limited

Printed at Media Centre, Blata l-Bajda, Malta

First published in 2005

ISBN 99932-672-2-8

Table of Contents

Author Profile

MR. ARTHUR FELICE, M.D., FRCS (ED) is a committed 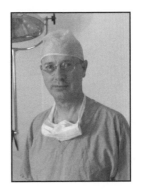 surgeon, married and has a daughter and a son. Born in Zabbar, Malta in 1947, he was educated at the local Government Primary School, the Lyceum and The University of Malta. He obtained his M.D. degree in 1971 and after working for two years at St. Luke's Hospital, Malta, furthered his surgical training at the Aberdeen and Inverness teaching hospitals. He passed his Final Fellowship exam at the Edinburgh College in 1975 and later moved to the St. George's Hospitals in London. On returning to Malta in late 1977, he was employed by the Health Department and the University. Between 1986 and 1988 he was Acting Head of Department of Surgery in both these institutions. He is presently Consultant Surgeon at St. Luke's Hospital and Senior Lecturer in Surgery at the University of Malta.

His publications range widely from Functional Somatic Syndromes to innovative treatment for Transitional Cell Carcinoma of the Urinary Bladder. The underlying note in all his work is a multidisciplinary approach to medical problems.

Acknowledgements

The late Mr William Owen, M.S., F.R.C.S., Consultant General Surgeon, Guy's and St. Thomas' Hospitals, London and Professor Mario Vassallo, B.A., Lic.D., D.Phil. (Oxon), Professor of Sociology, University of Malta and who both critically reviewed the original manuscipt of this book.

Elsevier Science for permission to draw on material from Surgical Decision Heinemann 1993.

Cambridge University Press for Permission to draw on material from 'The Technological Strategist' by Young, M.J., William, S.V. and Eisenberg, J.M. and 'Penetrating the Black Box' by Anbar, M., from The Machine at the Bedside eds Reiser, S.J. and Anbar, M. 1984.

My family who put up with me during the long gestation of this work.

Introduction

Quotation:

> Sir Karl Raimund Popper (1902 – 2001): Errors may lurk in our best theories. It is the responsibility of the professional to search for these errors.

For an undergraduate medical student, one of the most difficult and stressful periods is the transition from the pre-clinical to the clinical phase. Despite attempts at innovating the curriculum so as to smoothen the transition, there is still a distinct diversity in the way of thinking, attitudes as well as actions in these two phases of medical education, rendering the progress from one stage to the next difficult, if not traumatic.

The novices on the medical scene are showered with facts and data, which they can hardly appreciate or grasp let alone consume, assimilate and utilise. There is often no structured introduction to the various ways of clinical thinking, which eventually leads to logical clinical management. This is a real pity because an introduction to clinical methodology would surely help to streamline and not clutter the already overcrowded curriculum. A proper understanding of clinical methodology is bound to alter the educational environment in a way that medical students, and later on clinicians, will be more clear and serene in their problem solving and decision making. In time, they would be better equipped to confront and resolve the fundamental questions that arise in relation to their role inside and outside their profession. More importantly still, this will stimulate them to develop a good understanding of their own thoughts and actions.

The main purpose of this work is to address this very problem and to attempt to fill some of the lacunae in the interface between the pre-clinical and the clinical phase, in an attempt to overcome the considerable difficulties that result from this educational division. The delivery of this work was not easy and was preceded by a very long gestation. What follows is the result of long hours of teaching and reflection on teaching and clinical activity. Despite the fact that some views and methods that are proposed in subsequent pages may appear to be somewhat strongly presented, the emphasis is intentional. One can hardly be innovative by being neutral and seeking universal consensus at all costs.

In this book however, there is no attempt to be controversial for controversy's sake, or even forcibly original. Data and ideas expressed by other writers, from the medical and various other disciplines, have been referred to and duly acknowledged. It is hoped that the main contribution of this work results from the way this amalgam is used to explain, and hopefully improve, some aspects of the clinical process, in a way that can be appreciated by the medical student who has just ventured into the clinical scene.

The language used has been intentionally kept free from being overtly technical as a sign of acknowledgement that in contemporary society there exist many intelligent readers who are interested to know what members of other professions think about their work. Surgery, unfortunately perhaps, touches, at one time or another, practically all members of society, and the interest it provokes is therefore not surprising. This monograph constantly has this group of in mind, in the hope that this exercise in self-analysis contributes to a better understanding of surgery not only among the up and coming members of the profession itself, but also the public at large, which is fortunately becoming more interested in the ways surgeons think, decide and ultimately take decisions that affect their very life.

The clinical process could be compared with an extended detective story *(Plate 1)* and is similarly concerned with the restoration of order and what it takes to achieve this purpose. It is composed of three main phases which can be respectively called (a) the input; (b) the process itself and (c) the output. A brief introduction to each will set the scene for the later discussion.

Plate 1

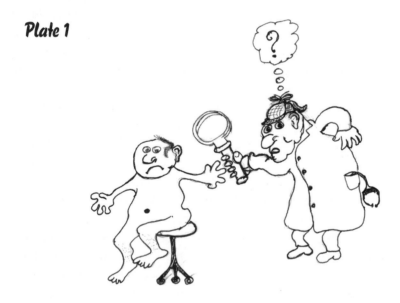

...the clinical process is like an extended detective story

The *input* refers to the situation involving the patient with the presenting complaint, shaded with his or her beliefs, fears, prejudices, pressures, psychological state, education, experience, information etc.

The *process* itself consists of clinical history taking, including history of the presenting complaint, systematic enquiry, past medical history, family history and social history; the physical examination eliciting positive or negative physical signs; special investigations of varying degrees of complexity, reliability, sensitivity, specificity and cost; diagnosis and treatment in its wider sense including follow-up, rehabilitation etc.

The *output* refers to the medical achievement which is often difficult to quantify *(Little, J.M)*.

The discussion in the coming chapters concerns methods, which could improve the *clinical process* itself.

The consultative, investigative and therapeutic methods in current use have evolved slowly over centuries and are used by innumerable clinicians worldwide. Is it appropriate, wise or useful to question these methods or at least some of their facets? There are, in fact signs of discontent coming from doctors and patients. Medical schools are making significant changes in the curricula in response to dissatisfaction with the way clinical experience and expertise is passed on to students. There are also statistical indications that the life of the 'medical learner' is by far too short to absorb the core knowledge base in its entirety by conventional methods. This aspect is treated at length in Chapter 4, which focuses on *Surgical Treatment*.

The introduction of new technologies in society has certainly improved our quality of life, but has also raised the level of concern about environmental causes of disease. Mobile phones, radio-frequency pollution and vaccines are frequently the subject of debate in relation to this. This concern may be, at least in part, justified and even potentially healthy. Its effects, however, have been extrapolated to a number of negative attitudes e.g. mistrust in the advice of health (and other) experts, a fervent belief in unproved 'natural' herbal remedies, a disenchantment with the health service in general and perhaps even an increase in psychosomatic manifestations *(Petrie, K.J., Wessely, S.)*.

Patients, consciously or subconsciously, often regard their diseases as defects and the clinical process as potentially involving degrading physical or psychological exposure. Their reaction often results in avoidance, silence, complaining or litigation *(Lazare, A.)*. Medical consumer groups criticise the medical profession for its impersonality, lack of empathy, poor communication and apparent self-interest. Medical insurance premiums are constantly on the rise, reflecting a higher incidence in malpractice claims (the cost of medical negligence in the British NHS rose by 7% in 1999) and general deterioration in relationship between the clinician and his patient. As a result, defensive medicine is increasingly adopted by clinicians and strategies of clinical risk management have evolved. Besides, the tightening of drug safety regulations (in itself a positive and well intentioned step forward but not without negative effects), medical care rationing disguised as reform, inappropriate and inadequate use of technology and the spiralling costs of healthcare have resulted in decreased respect for the medical profession amongst the public.

Training in surgery is in great part directed to form hypothesis and conceive questions, which can be answered by collecting data, but not so much to communicate. Clinicians are often not inclined to consider and admit the degree of reliability in their findings, predictions and procedures. It is important that the clinician is aware of the degree of certainty of the clinical process and, whenever it is possible and useful, this information should be shared with the patient and indeed, the public. Where the clinical process provides a high degree of certainty, it is possible to act in a mechanistic, logical manner. Guidelines and protocols are applicable and useful in such cases.

There are however, many clinical situations where such a degree of certainty does not obtain. These circumstances may be described as 'complex adaptive systems', i.e. a collection of individual factors with fuzzy boundaries, the effects of which are not entirely predictable and are interdependent. The detailed behaviour of this system is inherently non-linear and consequently unpredictable over a period of time. Only an overall pattern is predictable i.e. Attractor patterns *(Briggs, J.)*. To tackle such situations a clinician needs a degree of autonomy and flexibility, but he also needs to be plainly honest with his patients and the public. Many of the presumed deficiencies in health care are, in good part, attributable to unwillingness on the part of the public to accept the limits of effectiveness of medical management.

The shift of emphasis towards market-driven clinical enterprise has resulted in the measure of professional success being gauged according to financial success without limits, self-centered social accomplishments and title. This, together with the steadily progressive dominance of the biochemical aspects of clinical medicine and research, as well as the glorification of data obtained through the use of high technology at the expense of evidence-based good sense, are posing a serious threat to our concept of the good clinician. Core values cannot be divorced from clinical practice.

On the other hand, patients' expectations have increased, also as a result of partially informed media reports. All this has resulted in the soaring popularity of alternative medicine of all types, whilst doctors have become increasingly disillusioned or, at least, worried *(Le Fanu, J.)*. This disillusionment results from the altered relationship with employers, who impose targets and sometimes excessive controls, thus eroding the doctor's sphere of autonomy, declining doctor - patient relationship and also work-related problems such as high workload, stress, job insecurity and poor pay. Preparatory training for these new difficulties is not included in the medical curricula. Furthermore, the relationship of doctors with their employers and their patients begs for definition and a new equilibrium. Nearly half of all causes of morbidity in the USA, and probably in most other well developed countries, are linked to behavioural factors*(Editorial – The Lancet)*. Yet the behavioural and social content of formal medical training is insufficient. It is no longer surprising that doctors threaten and undertake strike action, whilst nurses leave the state health service and even their profession. Even though medical practitioners are often quoted by sociologists as constituting the almost perfect model of a profession, with all the autonomy of action that this has traditionally been understood to enjoy, increasingly, the stresses created by the need for doctors to work within large organizations are felt. Even top medical practitioners conducting cutting edge procedures in research oriented medical hospitals know that they cannot always implement what is technically possible because this might not always be consonant with what is financially feasible.

This scenario is complicated by the soaring cost of health in developed countries at a rate well beyond the rate of inflation, resulting in a bigger share of the total economy being necessary for health care. Governments in these countries react to these problems by attempting to control the steadily increasing cost of clinical medicine, measuring the cost-benefit of procedures (which is only to a degree applicable to clinical practice), and preaching best practice, audit and funding based on workload. Most of this audit and controls associated with it are well intentioned, but in part it is motivated by the lack of tolerance by politicians of any other group wielding any degree of power. The path ahead in such situations will probably involve a combination of strong central government (top-bottom) direction, for example through the enforcement of national or international standards, combined with powerful incentives for N.H.S. personnel to serve patients as efficiently as possible *(Enthoven, A.C.)*. One should encourage cooperation between the various government health bodies and perhaps, private enterprise (horizontal networks) to solve specific problems, *(Dixon, J., Preker, A.)* reaping the benefits of private sector efficiency.

Though one must guard against simplistic explanations and preconceived concepts, one has to admit that there are problems with the methods of the clinical process used at present, in many settings. Any attempt to define these problems and offer sensible alternatives is obviously justified, and therefore the answer to the rhetorical question proposed in the beginning of this introduction, is obviously in the affirmative.

How does this work propose to tackle the complex problems outlined above? The first four chapters deal with the different phases of the clinical process, emphasizing a utilitarian attitude in the methodology, with the intention of increasing efficiency, whilst accepting the essentially probabilistic nature of the process itself. Though the commercial environment pervasive in contemporary society cannot be eliminated, these chapters attempt to emphasize the value of more basic, and only apparently simpler, tools in medicine. The discussion focuses on the benefits derived from a properly taken clinical history and on a set of essential attitudes, such as correct use of logic and patient empathy. The purposeful alleviation of human suffering, rather than the obsessive collection of data or undue concentration on profit, is the focal point of this chapter. In this context, there is no attempt to belittle the importance of new technologies: their value is synthetically discussed and their proper application clearly indicated as an important aspect of wider and more holistic work ethos.

The following chapter deals with the various difficulties encountered in maintaining competence. These are discussed together with a set of suggested solutions and a balanced approach to new technologies. In the chapter that follows, medical research is treated from the point of view of the consumer who has to wade through mountains of new 'evidence' of variable quality and reliability. This chapter addresses the issues of validity and reliability in research to alert the consumers of medical research, be they medical students, specialist trainees, qualified clinicians or even interested members of the public, to the need to prune off the useless at an early stage, so as to be able to concentrate on what is relevant rather than be inundated with irrelevant trivia.

This approach entails constant reference to data from other disciplines, such as, philosophy, mathematics, the basic sciences, psychology, engineering, sociology, management studies and even the humanities. For those involved in the training of future clinicians, this side-expansion into so many areas during the training process might appear to be extravagant if not altogether irrelevant. It is hoped however that this monograph will demonstrate their useful application in tackling the above-mentioned issues. Indeed, it is strongly proposed throughout this work that the conventional divisions of knowledge, is not only artificial, but if strictly adhered to would inhibit cross-fertilization of ideas and slow down advancement. One can only overcome this through an 'open-mind' attitude and through constant encouragement of inter-professional communication and cooperation. The availability of networking on a scale previously unheard of, through the advances made in information technology, has made this clearly more possible than it had ever been dreamt of before. In their efforts to help present and future patients, clinicians need all the help they can get. More numerous and varied sources of knowledge do not inhibit, but rather help, the concentration of effort on particular problems and in their solution.

The main contribution of this monograph is to enrich the reader so that he can be better armed to face the pathological rogue. Having reflected on his own method, he acquires more knowledge. Being better aware of both his possibilities and his limitations should strengthen his intent to act decisively and promptly in the interest of his patients, whose trust rests solely on his efforts to save or improve the quality of their lives.

Chapter 1

Surgical Diagnosis

Quotation:
> Charles Darwin (1809 – 1882): 'How odd it is that anyone should not see that all observation must be for or against some view if it is to be of any service.'

The term *'Medicine'* is derived from *'Medix'* - an Etruscan word for a person who examined and adjudicated on local problems, sort of a local 'Justice of Peace' or Magistrate *(de Dombal, F.T.)*.

Sound practice of surgery requires the surgical 'magistrate' to possess:

- a detailed knowledge of the nature of disease,
- skills in diagnosis,
- the skills of helping the patient through his illness.

The definition of health by the WHO is 'complete physical, psychological and social wellbeing'. Professor Imre Loeffler remarked that this may perhaps be only achieved during simultaneous orgasm and would put us all in the unhealthy bracket for most of our time!

The standard definition of disease or abnormality as 'occurring when any measure is outside two standard deviations from the mean', is an amusing convention, since, given enough tests, all of us would at the end be found to have some abnormality.

There are two ways of conceiving 'disease' which actually constitute the two poles of a spectrum. The first is a 'Nominalist perspective' – a collection of abnormalities that appear to arise together, e.g. pernicious anaemia and the 'Essentialist perspective' – implying that signs and symptoms result from pathological processes which can be recognised and rectified e.g. appendicitis. *(Campbell, E.J., Roberts, R.S., Scadding, J.G.)*. Categories and concepts derive from our experience of the world *(ref. to 'Tailpiece')* and this also applies to such high level concepts as is 'disease'. *(Elstein, A.S.)*. There is more to a disease than a body mechanism which fails. The manner in which it effects the patient, the family and society is also important. The concept of disease is also subject to anthropological influences: What is considered as disease in one place may be regarded as a genetic abnormality, a crime or a sin in others e.g. alcoholism.

Patients present to their doctor with symptoms, which they suspect may be of a pathological nature. The frequency of this type of presentation is directly proportional to the life expectancy, level of health care and even levels of education in the region concerned *(Sen, A.)*. In part, this reflects the fact that in regions where serious diseases are common and dangers to life are high, a person is less likely to regard mild symptoms as worthy of complaint. The converse is also true. Where social conditions and levels of education are high, the media, including medical journalism and medical advertising, often encourage medicalisation and hypochondriasis. The boundaries between health, non-disease and disease, becomes blurred as a result. By 'non-diseases' one refers to fabricated diagnosis, universal effects e.g. aging, usual responses e.g. stretch marks, baldness, ends of spectrum and variants of normality, often wrongly regarded as pathological by patients and also some clinicians. One aspect of medicalisation is 'inventing diseases', creating markets for new products. Besides the non-diseases mentioned above, this also includes personal and social problems e.g. 'social phobia', 'female sexual dysfunction', risk factors described as diseases e.g. high serum cholesterol levels and osteoporosis.

Invented diseases:
(i)   Universal effects or ordinary processes or ailments of life e.g. wrinkles.
(ii) Mild symptoms portrayed as serious diseases e.g. IBS.
(iii) Social or personal problems presented as medical ones e.g. social phobia, alcoholism.
(iv) Risk factors presented as diseases e.g. osteoporosis, raised serum cholesterol levels.
(v)   Inflated incidence of disease so as to magnify its relative importance e.g. impotence, bone fractures caused by osteoporosis.
(vi) Ends of spectrum e.g. thigh fat pads, long noses, baldness.

Whichever the concept of disease and whatever the perspective, a clinician, just like a detective, has to develop, sharpen and improve his abilities for identifying and neutralizing the threatening rogue.

Traditionally, the good clinician has been regarded as possessing God-given or acquired powers of seeing further through a brick wall *(Hobsley, M.)*. The modern, popular view regards clinical acumen as proper application of modern health care technology, which will inevitably give you the right answers and therefore indicate the right treatment. If the first view was too romantic, the second is too simplistic. The commonly held concept of the doctor viewed as an omnipotent dispenser of health, may induce arrogance in some clinicians, but may also have rebound effects of an opposite nature on the public. Other factors, such as the modern attitude of regarding patients as problems to be tackled with maximal cost-benefit, the regarding of death as an enemy to be defeated at all costs and the consciousness (should we say the illusion) one's 'superior knowledge' may contribute to this arrogance on the part of clinicians. The antidote is the true knowledge of best evidence and the limitations thereof, as well as the realisation that doctors are only instruments of healing, nature being the real source. The characteristics of a good doctor include a combination of optimal skills and the sensitivity of the medical scientist with the intellectual capabilities of the medical humanist. When these are considered as part of a fallible human person, this ideal can only be considered as an approachable but unattainable chimera. We can only expect to have 'good enough' doctors.

If there are still brilliant and not so brilliant doctors – where lies the difference? It is often said that sharp principles for making clinical decisions are nearly impossible to define. This is a defeatist attitude. If we can define the method of diagnostic excellence, it should then be possible to instruct those to whom it is not inborn. Educational research indicates that good clinicians are better able to organise their minds to apply their knowledge to a particular problem, whether this is acquired in a formal manner or through experience. Generic reasoning skills do not feature prominently in the expert clinician's armamentarium. This, however, does not mean that formal training in reasoning skills would not result in a further improvement. Since the intention is to improve performance, rather than just concentrating on what is done correctly, it may be even more fruitful to focus on errors, which would lead to improvements. This should not be considered as a negative attitude. Errors help in the understanding of the diagnostic process just as the study of optical illusions help us understand the physiology and psychology of vision.

From psychology we learn that there are critical periods in the development of the mind during which input from the environment is necessary in order for specific functions to develop. This is called *Plasticity* – an interaction between the brain and the environment *(Elstein, A.S.)*. The trained mind is better equipped to tackle and solve problems, including clinical diagnostic problems. This may seem commonplace and predictable, but it is heartening to know that this has also been confirmed experimentally *(Rosen, M.P., Sands, D.Z., Morris, J., Drake, W., Davies, R.B.)*. This improved diagnostic ability goes beyond just avoiding irrational attitudes, which usually result from weakness of the will (i.e. acting against one's better judgement, wishful thinking, self deception, practising surgery of convenience etc.) What it entails is a more positive utilitarian attitude. One tries to analyse what are considered correct decisions and actions based on data collected, and one's criteria or beliefs, as well as the reasons for one's mistakes. The method can then be passed on, giving the learner a head-start in his quest for excellence. The central issue is how knowledge is initially learned, organised in memory and later accessed to solve problems. Problem solving and decision making are two separate processes in clinical reasoning.

Optimal decisions result from the application of a statistical decision-rule to data, as usually occurs in mathematics. Other methods are considered sub-optimal and this category includes surgical decision making *(Norman, G.R)*. Studying the strategies and biases in this field involves (i) the investigation of the mental processes and training of the successful clinician-diagnostician and (ii) the statistical association of clinical data and diseases. Expertise in clinical reasoning depends both on mastery of analytical rules or 'formal strategies' which involve the use of standard logical and statistical techniques leading to valid conclusions, and 'informal strategies' e.g. intuition, which involves rapid, automatic but learned (acquired) behaviour including judgements and decisions. In a clinical setting this is acquired through lengthy clinical training and accumulation of experience augmented by supervision and feedback *(Elstein, A.S.)*. One's very interpretation of external environment is moulded by previous experience, which is not necessarily dependent on expertise or seniority. This is not only a philosophical consideration *(Wittgenstein)* but has also been shown experimentally using illusions *(Deregowski, J.B)*. Furthermore, we learn from psychology that less than 5% of our sensory perceptions reach our consciousness, but all of them are deposited as more or less fixed engrams in the brain *(Habermann, E.)*. The definition of informal strategies proposed above is rather wide and would include pattern recognition e.g. in spot diagnosis and well assimilated algorithms. Such a wide definition of intuition is disputed by some authors *(Hobsley, M.)*, and this lack of standardisation has reduced the discussion on intuition to a semantic confusion.

Of course it takes more than the collection of good data, their evaluation, and the intellectual ability to channel these processes into the best possible action to make a good surgeon, though obviously, these are essential. A surgeon also needs the physical prowess and stamina to stand the strain of the amount of work needed to gain the necessary experience and dexterity in his (alas too short) lifetime, the aptitude, the dedication, the will to be critical and to learn at every opportunity, and the possession of good ethical values. In other words, the surgeon's attributes go beyond notions or knowledge into the realms of modality or the ability to deal with the patient. The satisfaction that one obtains, more than makes up for the sacrifice, effort and the inevitable disappointments involved in trying to attain these ends.

Diagnosis is opinion revision with imperfect information. Statistical decision theory involves ideal rationality under uncertainty but this does not translate well to the clinical scenario because of bias (refer to previous comments on the effect of experience and previously provided data on concepts and categories). Diagnostic reasoning has been explained by various psychological processes including, pattern recognition or categorisation, prototypes, practical reasoning, generating competing hypothesis (hypothesis testing) and algorithms *(Elstein, A.S.)*. In the clinical scenario, more than one of these methods may be used in tackling a single diagnostic problem. The most common problem solving approaches involve Hypothesis testing and Pattern recognition or Categorisation *(Elstein, A.S., Scwarz, A.)*.

An analogy can be made with the compound eye of insects: Imperfect and incomplete information from each small eye composing the compound eye, produces multiple, overlapping compound images, each component seen from a slightly different viewpoint *(Pulè, C.)*. This is elaborated by the insect brain to provide better information. Occasionally this information is still insufficient and the insect has to go round the object being examined to obtain better information. We use similar tactics in clinical diagnosis by utilising different mental processes and modalities.

Hypothesis Testing

In difficult diagnostic problems, one generates a number of hypotheses, indicating the additional features that would accompany each hypothesis if it were true. Further search for data is indicated by whichever hypothesis results as the strongest possibility i.e. the working hypothesis (working diagnosis) and those other hypothesis, which are rejected and therefore not followed up. Accuracy does not necessarily result from thoroughness when the latter is an obsessive collection of data for its own sake.

Pattern Recognition or Categorisation

This is more often useful in easy diagnostic problems. Its success depends more on mastery of the content than on strategy *(Patel, V.G., Groen, G.)*. Categorisation of the clinical picture is carried out by matching it to a specific case or cases experienced previously, or to an abstract prototype, which one has learnt through reading or other avenues of learning. The more complex and diversified the network of links between clinical features and diseases, syndromes and other clinical categories, the more is this method likely to be useful.

The traditional dogma of clinical method is that the clinician collects data from the patient in terms of (i) history, (ii) physical examination and (iii) special investigations. Thus, he builds a picture of the patient's clinical situation which he compares with his 'store of knowledge' thus arriving at a diagnosis.

One's knowledge is like an enormous book with a separate disease on each page, and one goes through these pages until one comes to the page that bears the closest resemblance to the clinical picture elicited from the patient. Medicine is a highly visual as well as intellectual discipline, which, in addition to studious observation, also relies on a process of 'pattern recognition ' and a personal template of 'health', from which departures and deviations are noted. This 'pattern recognition' of disease may be laborious but works in 'typical' cases, e.g. syndromes. However, at least a third of patients are not typical and the method of pattern recognition breaks down. Besides, in the acute situation, such laborious procedures are rarely practicable and short cuts have to be found.

The concept of a template of normality is not a simple consideration and is not necessarily synonymous with the average range: Thus if one considers bone density in ancestral bones, or other factors, such as blood pressure or serum cholesterol levels in isolated communities which follow a lifestyle typical of stone age communities, one realises that what we consider as average for western people, is not normal but actually high *(Law, M.R., Wald, N.J.)*.

The above-mentioned diagnostic processes may result in error through failure to generate the correct hypothesis, failure in data collection, or failure in interpretation of the collected data. Another practical and important consideration concerns the problem of the patient who is referred with a ready explicit diagnosis. In this situation, the clinician to whom the case has been referred may well undervalue any self-generated alternative diagnosis. The psychological reasons underlying this are not clear. They may include confirmation bias, in that one may tend to process the evidence in favour of the explicit diagnosis as a priority. This involves the search for new data as well as the memory recall of already collected data. Focusing on the explicitly presented diagnosis can make the interpretation of information in the light of self-generated diagnosis, more difficult. To prevent this bias one resorts to several strategies, which are here described *(Eva, K.V. et al.)*.

The 'short cuts' suggested in traditional teaching are:

a) The General Pathological Diagnosis *(Taxonomy)*.
i.e. the disease is congenital, inflammatory, traumatic, degenerative or neoplastic.

> e.g.: In an acute abdominal emergency one decides whether there is:
> (i)   obstruction of a hollow viscus,
> (ii)   peritoneal irritation due to inflammation, gangrene or perforation of an abdominal organ, or
> (iii) haemorrhage

One must note, however, that this taxonomic distinction between what is neoplastic, inflammatory and traumatic, may not be as clear-cut as previously assumed: Many inflammatory processes are notoriously pre-malignant e.g. ulcerative colitis and Marjolin's ulcer. Furthermore, inflammatory cells can be detected in cancers, deletion of cytokines and chemokines protects against experimental carcinogenesis and NSAIDs which are primarily anti-inflammatory, seem to reduce the incidence of various cancers e.g. of large intestine, oesophagus and stomach. Similarly low dose aspirin seems to decrease the recurrence rate of colonic adenomatous polyps.

b) The Differential Diagnosis.
i.e. a list of all possible conditions, (preferably in classified format), which might produce the patient's symptoms and signs. Special investigations then eliminate the possibilities in turn until the one-and-only diagnosis remains.

In fact surgical decision making falls into three phases:

1. Data collection
2. Data analysis
3. Decision as to patient management.

However surgical decisions are sometimes taken under conditions of considerable uncertainty. A proportion of such decisions may eventually prove to be imperfect though they may be based on the best available data at the time of decision taking. One may have to vary the sequence and emphasis of the three phases mentioned above. Usually junior doctors tend to collect a large amount of information, analyse it and then arrive at a decision, i.e. it is an approach by exhaustion (elimination) of possibilities. It may be considered an 'inductive reasoning process', that is, a process of collecting data in defence of a hypothesis, on the basis of similar data (history, physical signs and special investigations) leading to a similar diagnosis. The indiscriminate collection of all data in the way of a computer, is not, in my opinion, to be encouraged. Besides being wasteful, it may be misleading since one may collect information, which, besides being non-essential may also prove to be incorrect. One does realise, however, that one cannot be absolutely certain at every stage of the clinical process that a fact will necessarily be irrelevant to the clinical problem. It is also conceivable that such data may be found useful for research at a later date. In an era of cost-benefit analysis, however, such practices would not score very high!

The more experienced clinician adopts a goal-seeking (heuristic) attitude, asking a few relevant questions, forming a hypothesis (Hobsley calls it a 'Working Diagnosis') and then goes back to seek further information with which to confirm or refute this hypothesis. One develops, or adopts, short lists of important data, which allow decisions as to the 'next step'. For the use of the less experienced, data collection forms have been developed e.g. one referring to acute abdominal pain by the World Organisation of Gastroenterology. Such formal data collection forms are not necessarily complete, but are considered as containing important data by consensus of a number of experienced clinicians.

Clinical Thought Processes

The surgeon has traditionally combined the science and the art (in different proportions) and in the same way combines discursive (logical) reasoning and intuitive reasoning into a synthesis. This plays a role in diagnosis, choice in management including investigative approach, and in predicting outcomes. Unfortunately, intuitive reasoning suffers from several biases and there have been precious few studies investigating the effectiveness of clinical decision making based on intuitive thought. Heuristic reasoning is not synonymous with intuitive thought. Heuristic reasoning, which literally means aiming at discovery, aims at choosing correctly between alternative actions and is not primarily concerned with arriving at the truth. In a clinical setting this is done in the best interest of the patient. Formal clinical science, research and analysis improve the reliability of the premises, which are then channelled into utilitarian (goal-seeking) thought processes *(Gross, R., Lorenz, W.)*. In clinical situations characterised by uncertainty one uses both formal and informal strategies. As the proportion of 'certainties' becomes progressively more consistent, the need for intuitive thought (informal strategies) decreases; the science encroaches upon the art.

Though heuristic reasoning is often considered as a of hypothetico-deductive process of logic *(Black, D.A.K.)*, that is, a process whereby a hypothesis is formulated which is then subjected to rigorous testing, this is rather an application of Aristotelian 'Practical Reasoning', in contradistinction to theoretical reasoning. 'Intellect itself ..... moves nothing, but only the intellect which aims at an end is practical' *(Stumpf, S.E)*. The latter, i.e. theoretical reasoning, consists of a collection of true facts, which necessarily lead you to a conclusion. Practical reasoning leads to a logical action. It may be considered as a utilitarian approach i.e. finding the options to maximise utility. 'Concepts are not correct or incorrect they are more or less useful.' *(Wittgenstein, L.* – Philosophical Investigations).

Having emphasised the importance of 'Practical Reasoning' (or practical inference) in the clinical process, it is pertinent to explain further what is thereby meant: The importance of practical reasoning to human sciences has been compared to that of the deductive process in the natural sciences *(Ascombe, G.E.M.)*. The division of reasoning into 'theoretical' and 'practical' stems from Aristotle. Unfortunately later philosophers largely concentrated on theoretical reasoning, ignoring the latter. There where a few exceptions: Hegel, in his 'Logic', construed purposeful action as an inference, leading from the subjective setting of an end, through insight, into the objective connections of natural facts to the attainment of an end in action. (This concept had an impact even on Marxist thinking). Kant, in The Moral Law *(Paton, H.G.)*, said: 'Who wills the end, wills (so far as reason has a decisive influence on his actions) also the means which are indispensably necessary and in his power'. Wittgenstein has already been quoted previously. *(Von Wright)*.

The logical nature of practical reasoning is less clear than deductive, inductive or even hypothetico-deductive forms of theoretical reasoning. There is a difference of form between reasoning leading to action and reasoning for the truth of a conclusion. *(Ascombe, G.E.M.)*.

Basically, in practical reasoning, the first premises mentions an end to an action and the second premises some means to this end, e.g.

I want to attain end E.
To attain E, I must perform action A.
Therefore I should do A.

Here one should note that in this reasoning, action A is only a means of attaining end E and may not be compulsory. Other actions e.g. B, may also lead to E, as may be indicated by research evidence, Besides, carrying out A, in addition to the desired effect E, may also produce side-effect F. If B is found to attain E without side-effect F, the argument is altered accordingly.

The hallmark of practical reasoning is that the end is at a distance from the immediate action, the latter being the means to attain the end. The above were philosophical examples, which allow us to appreciate the application of practical reasoning to the following clinical situation:

I want to prevent this patient with right iliac fossa pain from developing peritonitis.

To achieve this I must explore or laparoscope this patient's abdomen, to make sure whether he has appendicitis and treat it.

Therefore prepare this patient for operation.

This is actually a chain of practical reasoning arguments, the conclusion of each providing the premises for the syllogism which follows *(Riolo, V.)*: RIF pain – diagnose appendicitis – decision to operate – treat appendicitis – prevent peritonitis.

It is clear that though it may be in the patient's interest to follow the above argument with the data in hand, the argument itself is not logically conclusive. For example, the right iliac fossa pain may be due to a cause that would not lead to peritonitis. Furthermore, the clinician concerned may not have the necessary expertise to order preparation for the procedure, confidently. Thus, the conclusion in practical reasoning is a declaration of intent, which is not necessarily true ore false, but is contingent and not logically necessary: In the above surgical example, the patient may be better off if the inexpert operator does not perform the procedure.

The following is another surgical example:

This patient who suffered blunt abdominal trauma, is in hypovolaemic shock from haemoperitneum.

To save his life I need to explore his abdomen surgically to stop the bleeding (whatever the source).

Therefore I shall perform a laparotomy.

The considerations directed at the previous example also apply, e.g. the clinician may help the patient more by resuscitating the patient and calling his senior.

Practical reasoning may either look to the past for motivations for previous actions (retrospective use), or to the future for actions (prospective use). In the retrospective application one starts from the conclusion and reconstructs the premises. This happens when we justify our actions:

The patient had to have urgent endotracheal intubation.

The patient had glottic spasm.

Patients with glottic spasm may be treated with endotracheal intubation.

In its prospective use, one sets out from the premises and the conclusion follows. Examples of this have been described earlier i.e. the examples referring to haemoperitoneum and RIF pain.

It is obvious to any clinician and especially to surgeons, that practical reasoning is used very frequently in clinical practice, though almost universally this is done without being conscious of the process. Obviously it is not the only process of logic that is applied clinically. In practice, the diagnostic process may involve any of several logical processes and perspectives *(Cox, K.)* e.g. inductive, deductive, hypothetico-deductive, and practical reasoning, as well as pattern recognition, heuristic application and priority setting in different degrees, with varying frequency and emphasis. Among these, practical reasoning, hypothetico-deductive logical processes and heuristic attitude together with cleaver prioritisation feature most prominently in the armamentarium of the good clinician.

Decision Making

Making a diagnosis means opinion revision with imperfect information. Applying Bayes' Theorem, the pre-test probability is either the known or presumed prevalence of the disease, before new information is acquired. The post-test probability is the probability of the disease after the new information is obtained. This depends on the pre-test probability and the strength of the evidence. The latter is often not easy to quantify and there are several possibilities of biases and errors e.g. clinicians tend to overestimate the probability of potentially serious but treatable diseases e.g. appendicitis, because they would hate to miss such a case.

The Clinical History

Going back to the traditional triad of history, physical examination and special investigations, one must appreciate the relative importance of these modalities.

Hampton et. al from Nottingham (1975) showed, in a very neat and important study, that in the vast majority of cases where a correct diagnosis is made, the diagnosis is already established or strongly suspected by the time the patient's history is taken. This had already been expressed by James Macenzie, a British physician, in his work published in 1920. He found that the patient's clinical history usually produced the earliest clues to the presence of disease and also furnished first hand evidence on how an organ functioned, providing a continuing index of the status and prognosis of disease *(Mackenzie, J.).* In a multinational study on the diagnostic value of symptoms and signs in 10,000 patients presenting with jaundice, doctors, relying only on clinical evidence, had an accuracy of 77%, whilst the diagnostic accuracy of a computer programme was 63% *(Lavelle, S.M. and Kavanagh, J.M.).* One experimentally proved factor which influences this comparative diagnostic accuracy is the doctor's level of experience *(Mc Adam, W.A.F., Brock, B., Armitage, T et al.), (de Dombal, Leaper, D.J., Horrocks, J.C.).* The clinician's intellectual effort to arrive at a correct diagnosis is another factor: In the diagnosis of acute abdominal pain, computer prediction can beat the inexperienced, unaided doctor by 10-20%, but when the same inexperienced doctors use the computer, their performance improves to match that of the computer *(Adams, D.H., Brooks, D.C.).* Yet other factors may influence diagnostic accuracy: these are related to the patient and his disease. The diagnosis of appendicitis is most difficult and is most likely to progress to perforation in the very young and the very old. The lesson to learn is that one should be more aggressive when dealing with patients in *this* age bracket. *(de Dombal, F.T.)*. The effect of time and level of expertise on diagnostic accuracy was investigated by de Dombal, Leaper and Horrocks and neatly expressed and tabulated as a percentage:

Level of expertise	1st 11 month period	2nd 8 month period
Diagnosis on admission	44.8%	38.9%
House-surgeons	72.2%	69.6%
Registrars	77.0%	82.1%
Senior clinician	79.6%	83.1%
Computer-aided system	91.8%	91.2%

There are two further things to note from the findings of this trial: The drop in accuracy referring to the admitting doctors and house-surgeons in the second period was probably the effect of increased data collection on inexperienced clinicians, which is a known phenomenon. Once the trial was over, the performance at all levels regressed back to the original levels. The trial itself, the novelty and the sense of competition played a part in the original improvement.

The importance of clinical history taking was emphasised by the advent of psychoanalysis and the introduction of medical social work by Richard Cabot in Massachusetts in the early twentieth century *(Cannon, I.M.)*. It is obvious that, whilst our senses and instruments can reveal many facts about a disease, only the patient can reveal how the illness affects him. Studies in Leeds by de Dombal et al. have confirmed this and we can all corroborate this (though unfortunately less scientifically) from our own experience. Furthermore, body organ systems are inter-related and influenced by the environment either directly or through psychological influences. Disregard of a proper clinical history, including the social history, may lead to failure of diagnosis and therapy. Clinical history taking entails more than following an outline and asking a standardised set of questions. In addition to developing an understanding of the patient and his disease, it makes the patient feel heard and understood. To obtain a healthy and fruitful doctor - patient relationship, the doctor must probe the hidden aspects of the patient's mind and not just his disease. This is done by careful observation and relevant questioning and by listening to the silences as well as the words. Data obtained while taking the clinical history, will indicate which aspects of this should be further explored in depth, suggesting the relevant systems or organs on which to focus the rest of the clinical process. This is an example of the heuristic attitude using practical reasoning as described previously. Looking at illness strictly from a cause and effect view, may miss out on the psychological influences that may effect symptoms and disease. The psycho - social history may suggest contributory factors in the patient's illness, help to evaluate the patient's sources of support, likely reactions to the disease and therapy, his coping mechanisms, strengths, concerns and phobias.

Unfortunately, this important point has become fogged by the modern technology explosion and history taking is not given its due importance in favour of reliance on the use and results of high technology. It is basic and very important to establish a good rapport with the patient, making sure that the latter understands the questions and that answers are interpreted correctly.

Language

Language exists on four levels *(Popper, K.R.)*:

1ˢᵗ level: Emotional or expressive, non-verbal e.g. scream or laughter.

2ⁿᵈ level: Appeals to the receiver for support, usually body language and non-verbal e.g. trembling and stammering from fear or excitement, an imploring look, etc.

3ʳᵈ level: descriptive - purely verbal.

4ᵗʰ level: argumentative requiring reciprocity.

Though in clinical history taking one is mostly using the third and fourth level, observing language levels one and two is often of considerable help in the clinical assessment. (What is new about 'narrative-based medicine'?!) The narrative nature of the history allows appreciation of the patient and his problem, but in order to focus more on the clinical problem, the extracted story is abstracted and translated into technical vocabulary. This may be incomprehensible to the patient but is important for standardisation of medical terminology and communication.

Having stressed the importance of the art of history taking, I must admit that there is an irritating problem with standardisation of terminology rendering the surgical interview vague or even misleading, e.g. 'sturdament', 'hass hażin', 'dwejjaq fuq l-istonku', 'hlewwa ta' qalb', 'bruda', 'hatfa', 'debbulizza', 'mohh' indicating both brain and frontal region, (maltese terminology often used by patients), also in English e.g. having a funny turn, dyspepsia, butterflies in the stomach, anorexia (quantitate), dementia, feeling out of sorts or unwell, taking a bad turn, vague terms meant to qualify and quantify pain e.g. dragging, dull, gnawing, lacerating, searing and suffering described in the language of pain (e.g. heartache, headache, pain and in the neck). Words indicating uncertainty, e.g.'Let's see what happens' or

'I think this might be....', may have a detrimental impact on the doctor - patient relationship and consequently on the whole clinical process. In an interesting article on doctor - patient communication *(Dobson, R.)*, the possibility of ambiguity in the use of the first person pronoun 'we' was studied: Doctors used 'we' on 24% of occasions while patients did so in only 2.9% of occasions. 'We' has an ambivalent meaning as either an inclusive 'you and I' or an exclusive 'we doctors and not patients'. Furthermore, the description of symptoms by the patient, may be influenced by his background or profession: an engineer may well colour his symptoms differently from an artist or even a labourer having the same physical symptoms. A depressive and a hypomaniac may express the same symptomatology in a diverse manner. A patient who has been cured of very serious disease and relieved of its troublesome symptoms, may then start complaining of minor symptoms previously disregarded. Besides, pain behaviour, which is in itself difficult to quantify and which may range from an account of a grimace to absenteeism from work may be included in the patients' account of his symptoms and their severity. This may be a source of further confusion.

It would be advantageous if, for a variety of clinical presentations one could delineate 'short lists' of symptoms in standardised terminology, which are crucial to particular diagnostic problems. The best example of this is the development of a common terminology for acute abdominal pain by the World Organisation of Gastroenterology referred to previously. Another laudable attempt in this direction is the International Prostate Symptom Score (I-PSS) adopted by the International Consensus Committee in 1994 (Chart 1.1). The symptom score is based on answers to seven questions concerning urinary symptoms designed for patient self-assessment. The answers are each assigned points from 0 to 5 and the patients can then be classified as having mild, moderate or severe symptoms. In general it is important to qualify and also quantify each symptom with regard to its location, quality, severity, timing, its setting, influencing factors and associated manifestations.

Even with this strategy there may be differences in the use and understanding of language by the doctor and the patient. Doctors and patients tend to speak in different languages: The former use medical terminology, objective description of symptoms expressed in physiological or biomedical terms. Patients tend to use non-technical terms indicating subjective descriptions of illness. This may lead to a serious breakdown of communication during the medical encounter, which may lead to adverse results. Clinician - patient communication involves:

1. Building a good doctor - patient relationship. *(Plate 2)*. This requires listening to the patient's story of the illness, guiding the discussion through the pathways of diagnostic reasoning. One becomes aware of the patient's concepts, feelings, beliefs and values in the process.

Chart 1.1 – *International Prostate Symptom Score.*

Patient name: _____   DOB: _____

ID: _____   Date of assessment:_____

Initial assessment ( ) Monitoring during _____

Therapy ( ) after _____   Therapy / Surgery ( ) _____

INTERNATIONAL PROSTATE SYMPTOM SCORE (I-PSS)						
	Not at all	Less than 1 time in 5	Less than half time	About half the time	More than half the time	Almost always
1. Over the past month, how often have you had a sensation of not emptying your bladder completely after you finished urinating?	0	1	2	3	4	5
2. Over the past month, how often have you had to urinate again less than two hours after you finished urinating?	0	1	2	3	4	5
3. Over the past month, how often have you stopped and started again several times when you urinated?	0	1	2	3	4	5
4. Over the past month, how often have you found it difficult to postpone urination?	0	1	2	3	4	5
5. Over the past month, how often have you had a weak urinary stream?	0	1	2	3	4	5
6. Over the past month, how often have you had to push or strain to begin urinating?	0	1	2	3	4	5
	None	1 time	2 times	3 times	4 times	5 or more times
7. Over the past month, how many times did you most typically get up to urinate from the time you went to bed at night until the time you got up in the morning?	0	1	2	3	4	5
Total I-PSS Score S=						
1. If you were to spend the rest of your life with your urinary condition just the way it is now, how would you feel about that?	Delighted	Pleased	Mostly satisfied	Mixed about equally satisfied and dissatisfied	Mostly dissatisfied	Unhappy	Terrible
Quality of life assessment index L=						

If available enter data for Q_{max} (cc/sec), R_{ml} (residual urine) and $V_{ml\,or\,gr}$ (prostate volume): S___ L___ Q___ R___ V___ (Code for R and V : **TA** = Transabdominal, **TR** = Transrectal Ultrasound, **MRI, CAT** = CT scan, **IVU, DRE** = Digital rectal examination, **END** = Endoscopy, **I&O** = Catheterisation, **X** = Other).

2. One opens the discussion, allowing the patient to complete her opening statement, encouraging her to talk about all her concerns.
3. Collecting information. This may involve open-ended or closed-ended questions as appropriate. One has to summarise, clarify and classify information, watching out for non-verbal messages.
4. Understand the patient's perspective which also includes taking a good social history.
5. Share the information, ensuring the mutual understanding of the terminology used on each side of the relationship.

Plate 2

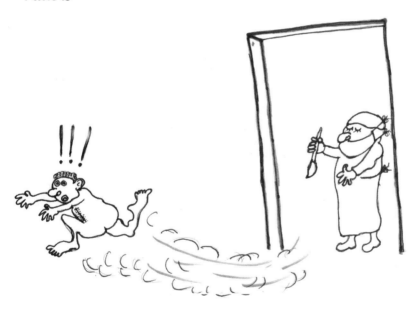

Building a good doctor-patient relationship

6. Reach an agreement regarding problems and plans, making sure that there are no other doubts or concerns and where relevant, one obtains the patient's documented consent *(Bayer – Fetzer Conference on Physician – Patient Communication).*

One may comment at this stage, that, since the solution of the clinical problem is of the highest priority for doctor and patient, understanding the pathological process is more important than an exhausting sympathetic attitude involving the personal problems of the patient, though these should not be ignored. In other words, though inquiry into the patient's social history and inner feelings is an integral and important part of history taking, it is not in the patient's interest for the clinician to become too involved. One should only get as much involved, as it serves to help the clinical relationship. An effort to implement this advice, should result in a favourable patient–doctor relationship and satisfaction, whilst improving clinical outcomes.

Clinical Information Standards

Problems of language involve the whole clinical process and are not limited to the clinical interview. Because of this, the concept of Clinical Information Standards has been developed. These consist of coding systems used for representing clinical concepts, in an attempt to ensure accuracy and consistency. These include three interdependent subtypes:

(a) Document structuring standards: Indicate the essential information that a particular clinical document must have e.g. a histopathology request form; an Accident and Emergency department admissions form; a death certificate.

(b) Term lexicon: Coded terms are explained and synonyms indicated e.g. Clinical Terms version 3; Snomed Clinical Terms.

(c) Ontologies: Medical knowledge is represented in a form that can be used by computers for clinical information systems and clinical decision support *(Gardner, M.)*.

One needs to ascertain which are the most efficient methods and resolve which bodies should assume control of these efforts.

The Physical Examination

The purpose of the clinical examination is:

(i) To confirm or refute hypothesis generated by the interview.

(ii) Provide evidence, i.e. possible causes, related to the patient's problems.

(iii) Provide evidence concerning the severity and extent of the disease.

(iv) Provide data for decisions on management e.g. general condition or fitness of the patient.

(v) May show coincidental pathology e.g. a patient presenting with bilateral inguinal hernia may turn out having chronic retention of urine, a carcinoma of the large bowel or any pathology causing a chronic cough.

One must note that at times the physical examination does not contribute any positive information, but even this, in itself may be useful. Regarding technique in general, one has to understand and correctly carry out the method leaving embarrassing or more painful signs till the end.

There is presently a tendency to denigrate the value of clinical signs. With the advent of sophisticated imaging techniques such as CT-Scanning, Ultrasonography, Nuclear Magnetic Resonance (NMR), Positron Emission Tomography and Gamma Camera, one may be led to conclude that one need not try to decide on the nature of an abdominal mass because the information obtained from these imaging techniques is far more detailed and (debatably) reliable. It must be remembered, however, that a sophisticated image is only an image to be interpreted subjectively, and is therefore prone to misinterpretation. This point will be discussed in more depth in a later chapter. When convincing clinical evidence does not tally with the results of special investigations, the clinician will then discuss the case with the imaging specialist and this dialogue may result in a revised opinion, repeated or alternative imaging.

The teaching of clinical skills is often delegated to instructors who are not the most experienced members of the team. This is even more dangerous when the students are just initiating their clinical training and may well result in the absorption of wrong techniques for eliciting signs, which are then carried over into clinical practice after qualification and registration. I shall not be singing the merits of all the classical physical signs we learn (or are supposed to learn) in our tutorials in Semeiotics. Certain signs have become hallowed by time and have been accepted as being reliable without ever being tested. Others have no clinical utility from the practical management view-point.

To give a practical example we shall discuss the value of clinical signs indicating whether an inguinal hernia is direct or indirect. The techniques suggested are neatly laid down in that wonderful textbook of clinical signs which is Hamilton Bailey's (by the way, students are well advised to know it from cover to cover and even backwards for it will influence the rest of their clinical life).

Briefly these are: (i)   the sign of the pubic bone
(ii)   the impingement tests
(iii) the inguinal occlusion test *(Clain, A.)*

Hobsley made a prospective trial using experienced clinicians to assess the above clinical signs and compared their assessment with findings at operation. In herniae that were proved at operation to be indirect, the observer was correct in 77% of cases. In similarly proved direct herniae, the observer was correct in only 59% of cases.

This shows that these signs are not very reliable even in experienced hands, (taking Kappa factor i.e. the relative frequency of the two types of herniae, into consideration).

In addition to this, one might argue that a pre-operative diagnosis of indirect or direct hernia is of no value whatsoever form the point of view of management. It does not influence the timing of the operation (direct herniae might also strangulate though less frequently), and does not influence the incision. When one makes the definite diagnosis at operation, one may then decide on the type of operative repair, accordingly. The fact that direct and indirect inguinal herniae follow different natural histories and that bilateral direct inguinal hernia are associated with other pathologies e.g. colonic malignancy or bladder outflow obstruction, is no argument in favour of relying on unreliable signs. So if we have clinical signs which are both inaccurate and useless, why do we continue to inflict them on students and patients alike?

When research provides us with sensitivity and specificity values for individual symptoms and signs for specific clinical conditions, *(refer to Ch.3 for definitions)*, the clinical assessment can take a more scientific course. An example of this is the work on acute appendicitis published independently by *Wagner et al.* and *Jahn et al.*:

Findings	Sensitivity	Specificity
Symptoms		
RIF pain	81%	53%
Anorexia	84%	66%
Nausea	58-68%	37-40%
Vomiting	49-51%	45-69%
Onset of pain before vomiting	100%	64%
Signs		
Fever	67%	69%
Guarding	39-74%	57-84%
Rebound tenderness	63%	69%
Rovsing's sign	68%	58%
Psoas sign	16%	95%

Even signs which are widely accepted as being diagnostically helpful, may be misinterpreted, even by the best clinicians. An assessment of auscultation findings of heart lesions by 900 physicians revealed that general physicians were correct in 41% of cases while heart specialists were correct in 79% of cases *(Scott Butterworth, J., Reppert, E.H.)*. The difference in the interpretation of signs is not due to sensory differences – clinicians essentially see and hear the same observations, but different criteria are used to interpret them. Standardisation of these criteria and the relevant training in their use improves the reliability of the sign.

Good technique in history taking, physical examination and the choice of investigation are dominated by the need to generate hypothesis quickly and to test them critically, rather than wasting time and money collecting information.

Special Investigations

This is the third source of data in the clinical process. The popular belief that data collected from this source, especially if backed by high technology and numerical values, provides us with the most exact, reliable and helpful data, is totally unfounded. The results of special investigations can occasionally be misleading.

For example, special investigations may indicate that a patient may have diverticular disease, hiatus hernia and cholelithiasis (Saint's Triad), when in fact the patient's symptoms are not caused by any of these. This topic will be elaborated in Chapter 3.

Assimilating and Assessing the Evidence

Accumulating data will not help unless it is properly digested and sorted out usefully. It has been demonstrated that the human mind, in contrast with the computer, looses diagnostic accuracy with increasing information *(de Dombal F.T. Horrocks, J.C., Staniland, J.R.)*. One has to ask several questions:

(i)   Is the information correct?
(ii)   What is the patient's problem?
(iii)   What is the likely disease category?
(iv)   What other diseases need consideration?
(v)   How severe is the disease or problem?
(vi)   Are there any other diseases or therapies, which may effect management?
(vii)   What is the next step in management?

To answer these questions in the process of clinical thinking, one identifies the abnormal findings, clusters these findings into logical groups, localises the data anatomically to organs or systems and when possible and interprets the findings in terms of the probable pathological, patho-physiological or psychosomatic process. Keeping in mind that one can only remember and evaluate about seven concepts at any one time when confronted with a problem *(de Dombal, F.T.)* and that data is not all of equal value. It is obvious that one must pin-point and use the information which is critical and useful i.e. adopt a goal-seeking (Heuristic) attitude. The aim should be to make the patient feel better, and not to make the doctor more self-assured with over enthusiastic use of data-collecting technology.

Uncertainty in Medicine

Since symptoms and signs are rarely typical, the approach is often necessarily 'probabilistic' i.e. evaluating balance of probabilities, rather than certainty. As a help in diagnosing such cases one may use;

a) The Clamp/Softley OMGE scoring system e.g. for Inflammatory Bowel Disease or Abdominal pain.
   or
b) The Bayes Theorem of
   (i)   *Prior probability* - what the odds are from general experience.
   (ii) *Conditional probability* - weight of new evidence alters the above.
   (iii) *Final probability* - There are no new items of evidence. Probability calculated.

An example to illustrate this, is the patient who presents with chest pain suggestive of myocardial infarction:

The prior probability from research evidence *(Weiner, D.A. et al.)* is 0.70. A positive exercise tolerance test raises the conditional probability to 0.88. Other evidence e.g. coronary angiography may push the final probability to higher levels.

Even with this 'help' one must accept a certain degree of uncertainty, which is inherent in surgical practice (the Probabilistic Paradigm in contradistinction to the Newtonian Mechanistic Paradigm) *(Bursztajn, H.J., Feinbloom, R., Hann, R., Brodstay, A.)*. This is not something to be ashamed of, or to hide. If patients were educated to the fact that medical science accepts uncertainty, this could form a basis for a better and more understanding patient-doctor relationship. This is a difficult concept to infuse into patients. However, overcoming the delusion of absolute medical certainty, by both surgeon and patient, will eventually lead to reduction of the uncertainty by making possible realistic decisions, which are understandable to both sides.

There is a very questionable tendency amongst doctors to regard a misdiagnosis in reading a healthy person as sick, as being less serious than missing the diagnosis in a sick person. This double standard is due to a difference in legal and professional consequences to the clinician. In fact, false positives are no greater help to the patient than false negatives. Training in evaluating clinical evidence is necessary to avoid pitfalls in interpreting data. It is this training and not the repetition of investigations, which can conceivably reduce the rate of misdiagnosis. An acceptable degree of precision of diagnostic test depends on three characteristics: the constancy of the phenomena being measured, the accuracy of the test and also the clinician's interpretation of these results. Developing expertise in evaluation of evidence is at least as important as all the other aids in diagnosis.

The Surgical Hypothesis (or Working Diagnosis)

This is often not a standard pathological term. It is a hypothesis on which the surgeon acts. It is no more than a resting place on the way to treatment. The rational decision-maker takes into account the probability of his working diagnosis, the utility and the consequences of his action or lack of action. He must maximise the utility of his actions. The surgical hypothesis may, and often is, altered at several stages in management of a case, in the light of new data as it emerges.

The diagnosis of 'Acute abdominal pain - cannot exclude appendicitis' means that one is not sure of the pathological diagnosis but it would be safer to urgently explore the abdomen surgically because of the dangers inherent in missing a possible or probable case of acute appendicitis.

Thus surgical hypothesis is not a static concept. It tells the surgeon what he should do at a specific moment, but does not claim to necessarily give perfect information. If, on exploration of the above patient, the surgeon discovers that the patient has e.g. A right tubal pregnancy and not appendicitis, he will then perform a right salpingectomy as well as an elective appendicectomy.

Though at times the Surgical Hypothesis may be the equivalent of a differential diagnosis, the heuristic (goal-seeking) tendency of the surgical hypothesis channels the thought of the surgeon in terms of what one should do for the patient rather than merely of what is wrong with patient. Thus the concept of the Surgical hypothesis lends itself to the construction of Management Pathways.

Examples of Management Pathways:

(i)   Scrotal Masses   See chart 2.3, 2.4 and 2.5 in chapter 2.

(ii) Breast Lumps   See charts 1.2, 1.3, 1.4 and 1.5 in this chapter.

(iii) Breast nipple discharge   See chart 1.6 in this chapter

These management pathways may look laborious but the sign of mastery of their use is really appreciated when one can forget them; or at least consult them only when going through difficult steps, i.e. when 'one's mind is not clear'.

While most clinicians will have a similar approach to these and other problems, they may disagree on certain steps in these pathways. They can then attempt to settle their differences either by argument or by a controlled trial.

Decision support systems will not, in the foreseeable future, replace surgical acumen or the concerned, dedicated and caring clinician, but available evidence suggests that symbiosis between computer and clinician is beneficial to the surgeon, the patient and the worried tax-payer. The effective use of modern technology by the surgeon is the only alternative to allowing oneself to become overwhelmed and destroyed in the resulting chaos.

This type of grounding must be combined with an ability to scientifically analyse and dissect our logical processes in surgical diagnosis and this should be borne in mind by those who so thoughtlessly eliminated the study of philosophy form the pre-medical curriculum. The introduction of such a discipline in the Sixth Form syllabus is laudable.

Diagnosing Psychosomatic Conditions

The interaction of psyche and soma will be discussed in more detail in Chapter 5. When symptoms and signs do not fit into known physiological, pathological or clinical pattern and the patient exhibits clear psychiatric symptoms in addition to the 'somatic' complaints, one is justified in suspecting a psychological aetiology. One must keep in mind however, that neurotic patients are not immune from getting physical illness and it is wise to adopt a double-track attitude, considering both the psychological and the somatic, well knowing that over-investigating neurotic patients may well aggravate their symptoms. Diagnosis of psychosomatic disease is thus, in great part, a positive process and not primarily one of exclusion of somatic disease. Detection of psychological influences, is important because untreated psychiatric pathology will inhibit response to conventional therapy for the somatic symptoms and may cause these patients to become 'chronic clinic attenders'.

Chart 1.2 – *Breast Lump (Hobsley, M., 1979)*

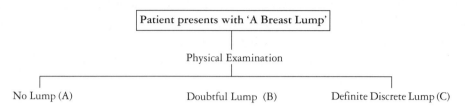

Chart 1.3 – *No Lump*

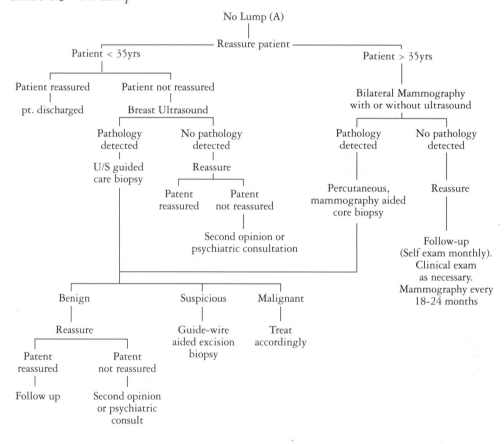

Chart 1.4 – *Doubtful Lump*

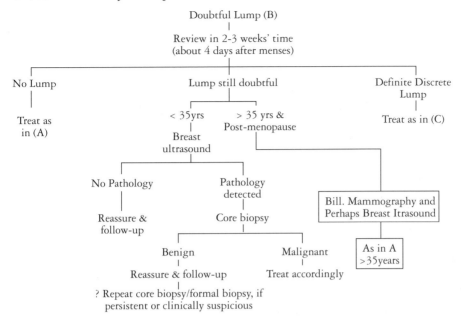

Chart 1.5 – *Definite Discrete Lump*

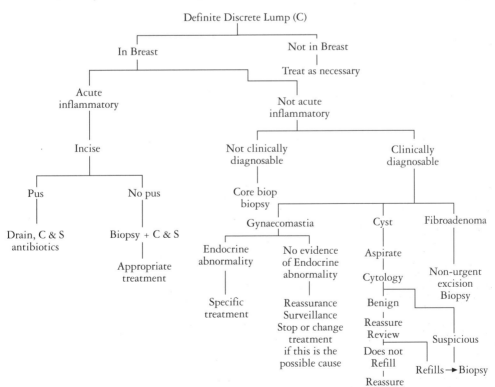

Chart 1.6 – *Spontaneous Nipple Discharge*

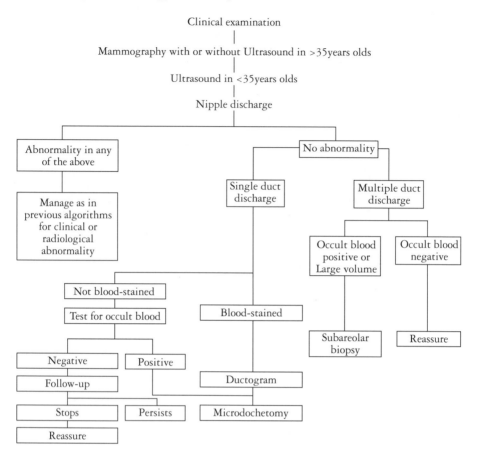

Documentation

An adequate medical record is one that enables the doctor to reconstruct the consultation without reference to memory.
This is essential:

1. To allow proper management decisions.
2. To record baseline observations of the patient's condition to be able to compare with future developments. ,
3. To communicate with others involved in the patient's care.
4. To provide data for medico-legal evidence if needed.
5. For research and teaching purposes.
6. For surgical audit *(Kyle, J.)*.

Interpretation of data, depends on a number of processes that are influenced by presentation and wording design, that is, the methods of entering data in the patient's notes and the design of laboratory report documents *(Wright, P., Jansen, C., Wyatt, J.C.)*. It is not very logical, for example, for Pathologists to insist, rightfully, on the entry of adequate clinical details on the request forms for histopathology, and then fail to include these same clinical details on their histopathology report, thus rendering its interpretation by the clinician, more difficult. Improved record design allows faster searches and more accurate interpretation of data, which in the long run will even reduce costs. There is a lot of room for improvement and consequently a fertile land for research as regards documentation design.

Evidence Based Medicine (EBM)

Good doctors use both individual clinical expertise and the best available clinical evidence in their practice. Neither of these factors is enough on its own. Without clinical expertise, even the best clinical evidence may be applied inappropriately; without the best clinical evidence, clinical practice becomes rapidly outdated.

Evidence-based medicine is a lifelong process of learning that creates a need for relevant information, the best way to obtain this information (clinical history, physical examination, special investigations, research results etc.), critically appraises this information (evidence) for validity and usefulness, applies this knowledge to clinical management and eventually evaluates the performance *(Sackett, D.L. et al.)*. Evidence based medicine attempts to apply statistical decision theory to clinical medicine.

Modern technology has rendered the application of EBM to clinical practice easier: These include new strategies for retrieving and appraising new evidence, systematic reviews e.g. the Cochrane collaboration, the publication of 'digests' of evidence, the application of information technology to evidence and the application of EBM to Continuous Medical Education, which is bound to increase the use of EBM with time. However, to date, evidence-based medicine skills are not well developed amongst clinicians. In fact it is not clear which of these skills are most conducive to improve the clinical encounter or patient outcomes. Research in this direction and more appropriate training could help to improve this state of affairs.

As with most things, EBM has its limitations; Evidence is often not clear or sufficiently concise. There may be difficulties in applying evidence to practice. EBM is often time consuming and needs training and skills of application. Finally one needs more evidence for the actual effectiveness of EBM in improving outcomes. The Fresno test is a valid performance based measure for the assessment of evidence based skills and of the effect of the introduction of teaching of EBM in medical education *(Ramor, K.D. et al.)*.

One also needs appropriate measures for the outputs in the NHS, which are of prime concern. The analysis of these findings, together with research data can then be synthesised into conclusions and recommendations, which can then be passed on to other health professionals, preferably indicating their estimated degree of

Diagnostic Errors *(Graber, M. et al.)*

Type	Reason	Example	Factors that reduce diagnostic error	Factors that cause persistence of diagnostic errors
No-fault error	Disease is silent, atypical or mimics something more common.	eg. Missed colonic cancer in a patient who refused opportunistic screening.	Advances in medical knowledge aids, diagnostic aids and technology.	(i) The probabilistic nature of clinical diagnosis and the inherent fallibility of the human mind. (ii) The emergence of new diseases. (iii) Non-compliant patients. (iv) Limitations of diagnostic aids.
Systems error	Latent imperfections in the health care system.	eg. Diagnosis missed by trainees.	Systems improvement.	(i) The limitation of resources with resulting tradeoffs. (ii) Changes create new possibilities for error. (iii) Improvements lag behind the emergence of error.
Cognitive error	(i) Deficient core knowledge. (ii) Faulty data collection. (iii) Faulty data analysis. (iv) Poor logic.	eg. Missing a breast carcinoma relying only on imaging and failing to perform an adequate clinical examination.	(i) Improving standards of basic knowledge and clinical reasoning. (ii) Second opinions. (iii) Decision support systems. (iv) Guidelines and algorithms. (v) Easy access to consultation.	(i) Limitations of the human cognitive process. (ii) Limitations of intuitive thought. (iii) Biases.

accuracy. This should influence policy makers to produce health policies consistent with valid research evidence, and similarly to managers to ensure cost-effective practice, clinicians to apply this to day-to-day patient care and users to influence health care choices in a logical manner. Unfortunately, health managers often use the expression 'there is no evidence' when they really mean 'we cannot afford it'. Scientific evidence is not present or absent, but needs to be sought, interpreted, extrapolated and integrated, before one can reach any practical conclusion as to its applicability.

Conclusive Remark

One should favour an educational system, which is better able to respond to changes in the outside world by teaching scientific behaviour as well as scientific facts, adapting to the changing doctor - patient relationship, promoting multiprofessional teamwork and teaching techniques involving team work. In practice, this should reflect the changing pattern of disease and health care delivery, promote the use of information technology and give priority to training in problem solving.

Methodology must form part of the surgical curriculum and should have an interdisciplinary basis with surgeons, philosophers, psychologists, information technologists, mathematicians and perhaps even social scientists taking part, in an integrated manner, using strictly surgical (medical) examples. The experience and training of other professional groups, even outside the health sector, is often illuminating and helpful in our search for the advancement of surgical practice.

All this, in addition to the advances in medical science and technology, as well as systems improvement, should lead to a steady improvement in the degree and rate of diagnostic error, though one cannot expect to eliminate it.

Chapter 2

Aids to Patient Management

Quotation:

> The London Times 1834, commenting on Laennec's introduction of the stethoscope: 'That it will ever come into general use notwithstanding its value, is extremely doubtful; because its beneficial application requires much time and gives a good bit of trouble to the patient and practitioner.'

The conscious attempt to make best use of current evidence in making clinical decisions is hardly new. It has been given several names, the latest and most fashionable being Evidence-base Medicine and Decision Science. Basically this entails the integration of individual clinical expertise with the best available clinical evidence from systematic research. These two factors are complementary and not exclusive. The selection of appropriate actions from a wide spectrum of possibilities, balancing trade-offs between desirables and non- desirables, is one of the basic skills in clinical practice. Thus, any formal method deigned to evaluate and aid in this decision making would be both desirable and important.

In making any decision one defines the problem, specifies alternative actions and then determines possible outcomes from each alternative action. Clinical decision making is based on different degrees of evidence, values or preferences and circumstances. Furthermore, decision making is necessarily influenced by bias, which is due to the direction from which we see things. Decision Science focuses on recognition and accounting for biases and thus involves individual decisions. Evidence-based Medicine involves evaluating information and using this digested and selected data for decision making, in an attempt to make this more scientific and legitimate. It rests on the choice of accepting other people's research results and judgements. The disadvantage of EBM is its rigidity. Both these tools are valuable supports for medical decision making and should be used in synergy *(Schulkin, J.)*.

Several methods of deciding on diagnostic and therapeutic strategies have been proposed.

These include:

1. Multivariate analysis (equations)
2. Decision analysis including Objective Medical Decision making (OMDM)
3. Patient data banks
4. Information Technology and Artificial intelligence
5. Clinical Problem Analysis
6. Mechanistic Case Diagramming and
7. Clinical Algorithms.

These aids to decision making presuppose a mind with unlimited reasoning powers, computing intricate probabilities, utilities or weigh scales. Another suggested alternative is to utilise the concept of a limited mind using a toolbox of fast and frugal heuristics i.e. rules of thumb *(Girgenza, G., Todd, P.)*. This latter method may be applied as 'satisficing' i.e. searching through a list of available alternatives, or, where little information and computation is used in decision making, as fast and frugal heuristics *(Elwyn, G., Edwards, A., Eccles, M., Rovner, D.)*. The trade-off between accuracy and fast frugality is actual and central in the practical clinical situation where time and resources are limited.

A general strategy applicable to a wide range of clinical situations would be useful to help clinicians in decision-making avoiding inconsistencies and, hopefully, mistakes. Evidence-based Medicine and Decision Analysis, both help in quantifying evidence, taking into account uncertainties and systematically weighing advantages and risks of alternative treatment strategies. Multivariate equations and Decision analysis are rather complex and difficult to master. Others, like Patient data banks and Artificial intelligence are being introduced in our patient-doctor set-up. Objective Medical Decision making may be of help, but does not eliminate the difficulties of clinical reality e.g. insufficient or faulty data.

Multivariate Analysis

This allows simultaneous considerations of multiple factors, each factor having a different degree of importance for the decision. Relevant variables are identified and weighted differently. A mathematical model is then developed using complex mathematics and computer technology. The mathematical equation can then be applied to decide on diagnostic or therapeutic methodology.

Advantages: (i) Can evaluate information consistently and quantitatively.

(ii) May lead to better use of resources by limiting hospital admissions and allowing better use of technology.

Limitations: (i) The patients on whom it is applied may be different from the ones used in developing the model.

(ii) The variables used for analysis may be poorly defined or selected.

(iii) The weighting given to variables is subjective.

Decision Analysis

In Decision Analysis, the decision making process is laid out in the form of a branching tree, with decisions represented as square nodes, the chances of an outcome as circular nodes and the passage of time as lines. The different node shapes are in fact just conventions, which add little to the discussion on the possible clinical application of the technique. In Formal Decision Analysis, one assesses the (a) probability of an outcome and (b) the utility i.e. the subjective worth of an outcome of a surgical decision, to the patient. A mathematical value (usually a scale from 0 to 1) is assigned to this.

Clinical Problem Analysis

This is more than just a diagnostic method, but proposes a systematic way for resolving a clinical problem in its entirety. It involves:

(i) Drawing a list of the patient's problems obtained through history taking, observation and physical examination.

(ii) Pointing out the relevant physical findings.

(iii) Attempting to explain the findings in terms of pathophysiology and anatomy.

(iv) Constructing an action plan which includes:

    a. Indicating further data collection from special investigations.

    b. Therapeutic action involving prevention, therapy, follow-up and rehabilitation. *(Custers, E.J., Stuyt, P.M., De Vries Robbi, P.)*

Mechanistic Case Diagramming

The approach is similar to Clinical Problem Analysis and to the 'aetiological algorithm' *(Engelberg, J.)*. It traces in a stepwise form the pathophysiologcal mechanisms resulting from the underlying causes of disease, to clinical symptoms and signs, as well as the various consequences and complications of the disease. It encourages the understanding of the symptomatology and a holistic approach to disease since various aetiological factors, including psychological ones, may be included in the diagram. This method also encourages interdisciplinary integration of knowledge and allows scrutiny and critical appraisal of the logic used in a particular clinical process. It is a useful tool for problem-based learning and once the technique has been well assimilated, it may be easily and profitably applied to new clinical situations. The following is an example of a Mechanistic Case Diagram applied to a case of intestinal obstruction:

Mechanistic case diagram applied to a case of intestinal obstruction

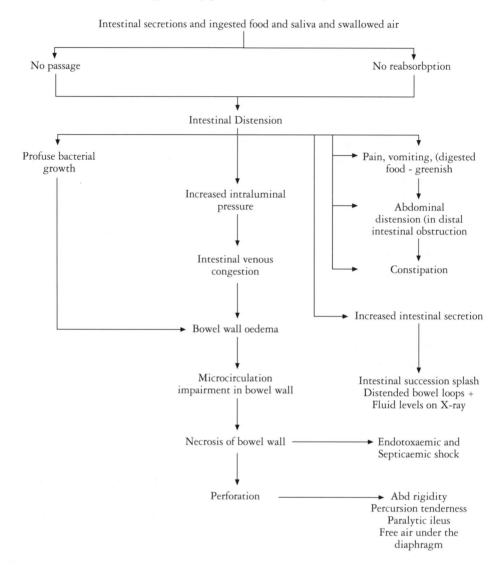

The Clinical Algorithm

This is an easy to learn, easily applied method *(Plate 3)* that assists the clinician in pursuing a logical, step-by-step evaluation and management plan. Such management pathways, (e.g. Clinical Algorithms), may be used: (i). to indicate protocols for management of specific clinical problems (ii). to guide paramedical staff in the management of common problems (iii). to evaluate the quality of care that has been provided. This method should not be interpreted as an attempt to aid the cost-cutters or to suppress clinical freedom. Pursuing the useless may constitute an expression of freedom but is also clinical nonsense. Indicating pathways, which identify and apply the most efficacious management to maximise the quality and quantity of life of individual patients may result, both in increased or in decreased cost, of health care. In general terms, the aims of this method are:

a. To generate a working hypothesis at an early stage.
b. To avoid excessive data gathering, including superfluous investigative procedures.
c. To avoid erroneous interpretation of data.
d. To encourage hypothesis testing leading to confirming or discarding the hypothesis. Thus one keeps an open mind, in a true Popperian scientific tradition, hopefully avoiding confirmation bias.

Plate 3

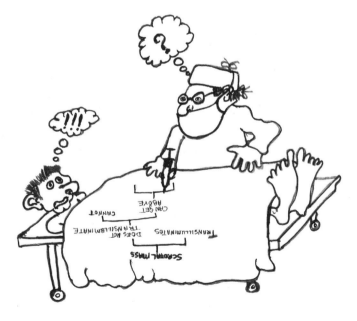

The clinical algorithm is an easily applied method...

History

1800 BC: Babylonian mathematicians set step-by-step rules to solve many types of equations.

825 AD: Persian mathematician Al-Khowarizmi (thus Algorithm) wrote a classical textbook on arithmetic.

Early 1970's: Clinical scientists at Harvard and Dartmouth Universities apply Algorithms to medical problems.

Definition

The Algorithm is a branching logic flowchart that leads the practitioner through the necessary steps in management, depending on the presence of certain findings or the occurrence of certain events. It is applicable to any practical discipline. Algorithms have been used in industry far before they were consciously applied to medicine (like a lot of other technologies). An example is Chart 2.1 - the problem of a non-starting engine, for the benefit of the more technically minded. A clinical algorithm thus indicates the components of history and physical examination that are needed, and the diagnostic tests that should be obtained. It is different from a decision tree in that the latter is probabilistic (i.e. it provides probabilities that certain events may happen at chance nodes, and then the clinician makes his decisions based on this).An 'algorithm' is not synonymous with a 'flow chart'. A clinical algorithm is a step-by-step approach to solving a clinical problem involving logic. A flow chart is a graphic format showing linked, sequential events over time. Thus flow charts may depict the flow of historical events (historical flow charts – e.g. Chart 2.2), the flow of physical events (e.g. the coagulation cascade), or the flow of dependent decisions (e.g. the clinical algorithm or the decision tree). The innumerable clinical guidelines which fill our mail-boxes are often an expression of the latter type of algorithm. To be useful, the authors of such algorithms have to identify the major decision points and their consequences, to point out the necessary evidence for valid decisions on individual patients, and present the decisions in a concise, accessible and easily applicable layout.

Chart 2.1 – *The use of an algorithm to diagnose a non-start fault (Pulè, C.)*

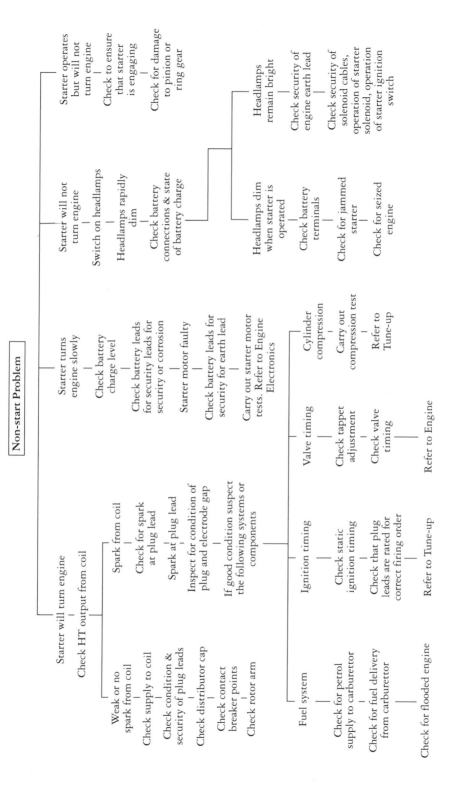

Chart 2.2 – *Stages of hepartitis B disease (* symptomatic, ** asymptomatic) (1998)*

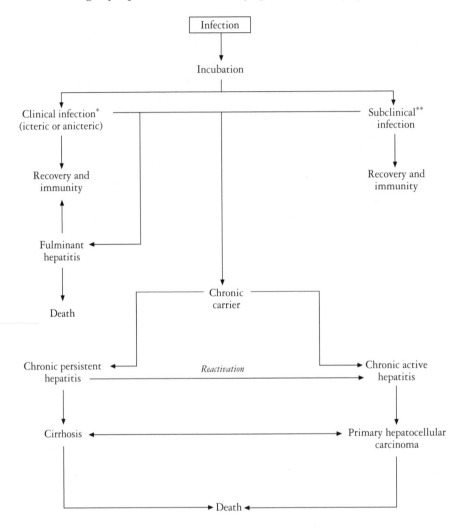

Decision Analysis

The following is an example of a decision tree applied to coronary artery disease indicating the probabilities of subsequent disease:

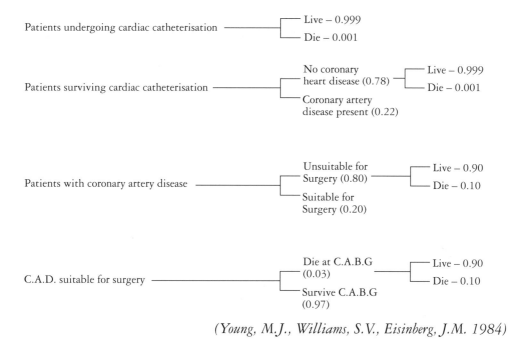

(Young, M.J., Williams, S.V., Eisinberg, J.M. 1984)

When Decision Analysis is applied to a decision tree, one also includes the concept of utility, meaning that one quantifies a value assigned to each outcome. Utilities may be objective e.g. costs, survival rates. On the other hand, they may be subjective when a value (0 to 1 or 0 to 100) is assigned in an arbitrary or semi-arbitrary manner using the lottery technique or game theory. (Dawson, B., Trapp, R.G.).

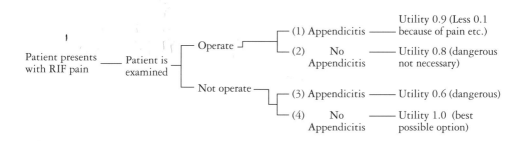

The following is an example applied to RIF pain:

When one evaluates the decision tree regarding coronary artery diseases, one concludes that a decision to perform cardiac catheterisation with a plan to operate on suitable (defined) patients, provides greater survival than a decision not to perform cardiac catheterisation. Also the best possible option for the second decision tree would be not to have appendicitis and not to be operated, while the second best (because of post-op pain, possible complications, etc.) is to have an appendicectomy if one does have appendicitis.

The test of robustness for decision analysis is called sensitivity analysis. This involves changing the estimates for probability and utility, and one sees whether the decision changes on analysis. The utility of a decision or of operative outcome (UOP) is the sum of the utilities of the two possible outcomes multiplied in each case by the probability of that outcome occurring.

$$UOP = Pa_1U_1 + (1-Pa_1)U_2$$

This utility assessment refers to utility to the patients. Though this may sound commonplace, one should realise that this may well be different from the utility referring to the public or to the doctor. E.g. a patient suffering from AIDS needing operative therapy.

If one constructs a graph for the above equation expressing utility to patient against probability of appendicitis in the two options i.e. (a) With operation (b) Without operation, the following distribution is obtained.

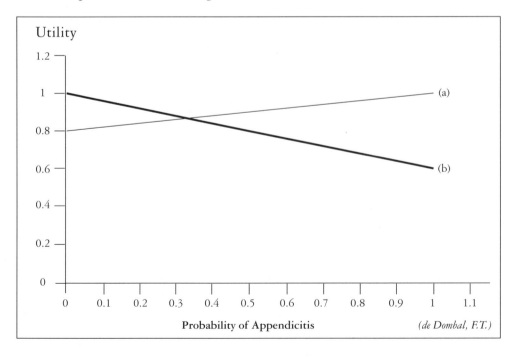

(de Dombal, F.T.)

If the two linear graphs were not to cross, then one choice is always better than the other and would become the preferred method in all circumstances. When the two graphs cross as in the case of appendicitis, then the intersection of the two graphs shows that when the probability of appendicitis is equal or more than 0.4 (i.e. 40% chance) one would do better to operate. This is called the Threshold or Point of Indifference for the two options in the case of appendicitis - at this point one option is not better or worse than the other. Above this probability the utility of operation is more than withholding operative therapy. Thus, the threshold is the end of the indication for one option and the beginning of the indication for another. At threshold, extra data should be obtained unless the 'cost' of getting this information offsets the potential advantages.

This method could be applied to other surgical problems:

For example one could consider applying Decision Analysis to the problem of exploring (or otherwise) the common bile duct during cholecystectomy:

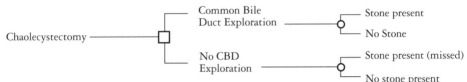

One could plot graphs of the expected utilities of the two options against the probability of the stone occurring, varying the values for the probability of stone occurrence:

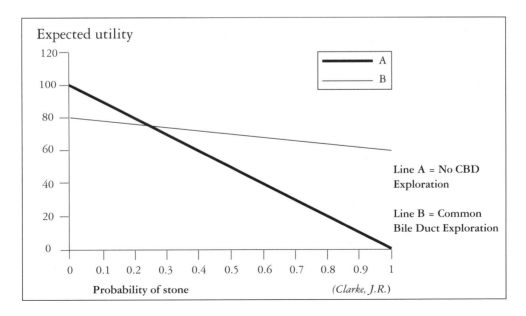

Note that the utility to the patient decreases with increasing probability of CBD stone even when CBD exploration is performed, because having a CBD stone is always an adverse factor.

The point at which the two graphs intersect is the Threshold. This is the value of a factor, in this case the probability of stone, at which one option stops being the better choice and the other option becomes advisable. i.e. 0.26 probability of CBD stone.

The probability may be revised if there is additional data e.g. raised WBC count in the case of appendicitis, or positive per-operative cholangiogram or ultrasonography in the case of CBD stone.

Decision analysis may be used to compare different methods of investigation as well as treatment:

The most effective protocol for screening asymptomatic patients for carcinoma of the colon has been investigated in this way *(Brandeau, M.L., Eddy, D.M.)*. The results are both interesting and useful. Performing a Barium enema prior to colonoscopy or sigmoidoscopy increases the overall sensitivity for cancerous or pre-cancerous lesions by only 0.3% but increases the cost by about 45 USD. Using the Barium enema as a screening procedure and following it up with a colonoscopy in suspicious cases only reduces the pickup rate by only 2% but results in a reduction in costs of 165 USD. Colonoscopy on its own reduces the pickup rate from 90% to 80%. Repeated faecal occult blood testing is not sufficiently effective with a false negative rate of 45%.

Though apparently attractive, it is not difficult to imagine why such formal utility assessment is not normally carried out in the clinical scenario: it is not practical, clinicians are not often trained in the technique, it is also time consuming and stressful for both doctor and patient, who may not be in the right mind for such an exercise *(Weinstein, M.C., Feneberg, H.V.)*. The results of decision analysis in clinical research, may however, provide best evidence that may help in making clinical decisions.

Advantages of Formal Decision Analysis
1. It offers a systematic approach to decision making based on rationality.
2. Can incorporate many factors.
3. It is based on a fuller range of information than is possible in an unstructured approach.
4. It acknowledges choices and uncertainties.
5. Potentially enhances patient participation in decision making through the consideration of patient utility even at individual level. This avoids the contradiction of 'average preference'.
6. Balances harms and benefits considering best evidence and patient utility in a situation of complex outcomes.

7. Allows the inclusion of specific aspects including economic ones, local complication rates and local availability into the equation.

Problems with Formal Decision Analysis

1. Typical patients are not so common.
2. Standardisation of decision analysis goes against individualisation of patient care, though individual level decision analysis corrects this.
3. Outcome data used in decision analysis may not reflect the risk to an individual or even a specific population. For example, the outcome or utility values for appendicitis may not reflect those of appendicitis in pregnancy or when accompanied by some other disease. Clinical heterogenicity is a limitation for the use of this technique.
4. Families of outcomes cannot always be disentangled and weighted separately.
5. Utilities assigned to each outcome are, at best, educated guesses and hardly definite.
6. There is difficulty in expressing patients' feelings in numerical terms e.g. with respect to pain, quality of life, patient satisfaction.
7. Practical application of clinical decision analysis would require longer consultations, re-scheduled appointments and increased staff requirements.
8. Data on which decision trees are based may become superseded, e.g. the decision tree data on cardiac catheterisation and CABG quoted earlier, are surely superseded due to improvements in the technique.
9. Decision making often involves other factors than just maximisation of utilities.
10. Application of decision analysis to the clinical situation does not necessarily lead to better decisions. The results of such an exercise should not be regarded as a dictat, but rather as one more piece of evidence in the clinical situation. It should help us think rather than stop us from thinking.

Algorithms

In contrast, a Clinical Algorithm shows what should be done in the event of a certain clinical situation. No probabilities are expressed and usually the management is indicated without choice of alternatives for the specific clinical event.

It is advisable that both algorithms and decision trees, are dated so that whoever uses them is aware of any possibility that the data on which they are based has become superseded.

Examples of Clinical Algorithms:

A. Scrotal Swellings - Charts 2.3, 2.4, and 2.5 (1979).
B. Management of Burns - Chart 2.6 (1987).
C. Haematuria - Chart 2.7 (1995).
D. Management of Transitional cell Carcinoma of the Urinary Bladder - Chart 2.8. (1996).

Chart 2.3 – *Scrotal Swelling*

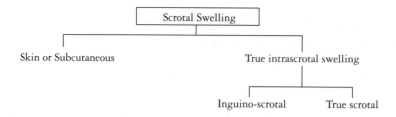

Chart 2.4 – *Inguino-scrotal Swelling*

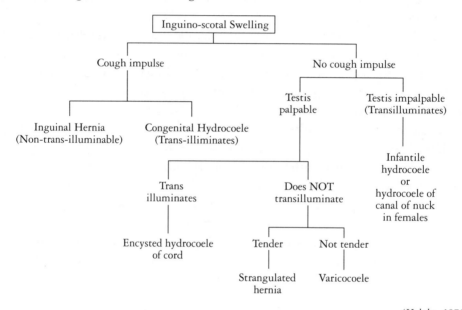

(Hobsley, 1979)

Chart 2.5 – *True Scrotal Swelling*

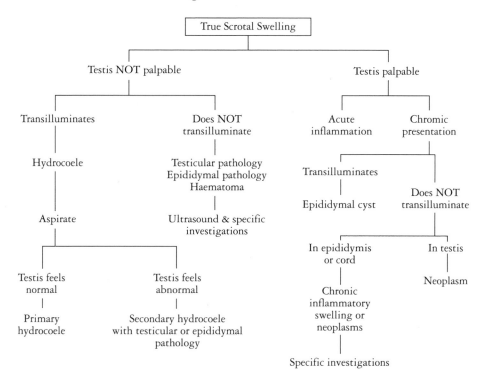

(Adapted from Hobsley, 1979)

Chart 2.6 – *Burns (1987)*

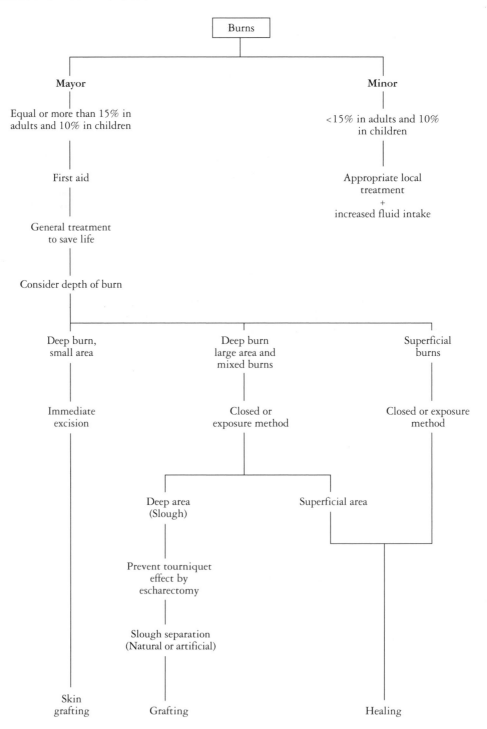

Chart 2.7 - *Haematuria (1995)*

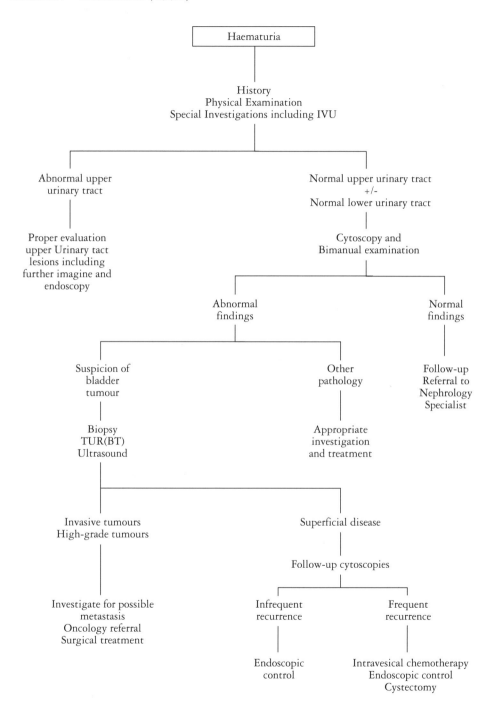

Chart 2.8 - *Management of Transitional Cell Carcinoma of The Bladder (1996)*

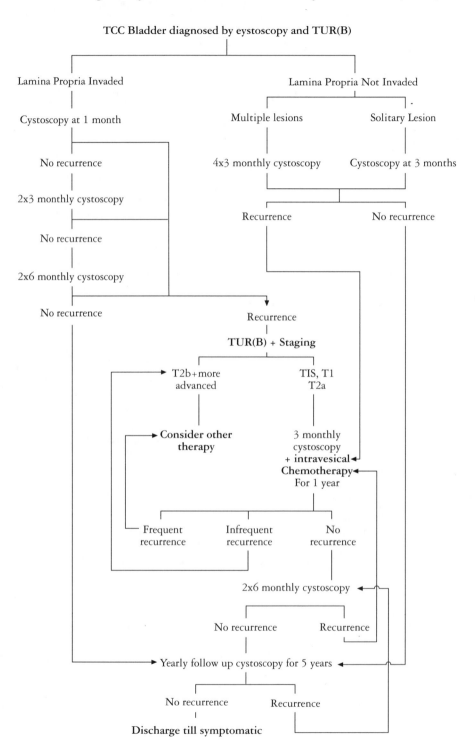

Chart 2.9 *Management of Right Lower Quadrant Abdominal Pain*

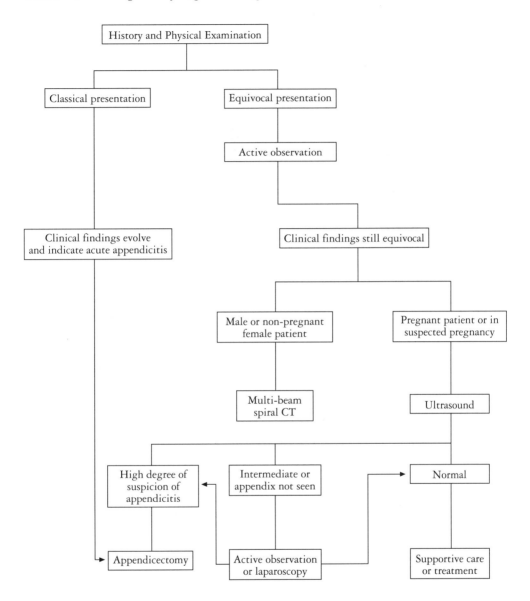

N.B. The clinical branches of this algorithm, on their own, can result in a negative appendicitis rate of 4-8% *(Jones, P.F., Krukowski, Z.H., Youngson, G.G.)*. The imaging branch of the algorithm is used in a minority of cases, though this is debatable *(Paulson, E.K. et al.)*.

Utility of Algorithms

Many clinicians think that the common clinical problems to which Algorithms are applicable are too simple to require any form of aid to decision making. It is difficult to agree with this view for several reasons:

a. Common clinical problems are rarely 'simple'.

b. Medical decision making may be flawed because of a variety of subjective and objective causes.

c. The algorithm defines the clinical data to be collected on an individual patient with the particular problem, thus reducing wastage of clinician's time and effort.

d. Algorithms define the clinical findings that should lead to particular special investigations thus avoiding unnecessary expense.

e. They occasionally define criteria for obtaining consultation with a particular specialist.

f. Algorithms define the clinical findings leading to specific management.

g. They induce the clinical scientist to analyse and dissect his thought processes in the management of his patients when he is planning the Algorithms.

h. Algorithmic criteria yield a stepwise increase of information and specification on the clinical problem, which is superior to assessment based on lists of criteria.

i. Clinical algorithms may be used to assess the quality of care:
E.g. one can compare different management pathways (algorithms) to assess the best protocol to follow.

j. With the use of advanced technologies e.g. Personal computers etc. patients may be able to gain access to authoritative medical databases, and for common medical problems, use algorithms available on line to diagnose and perhaps treat themselves. This may be one aspect of future changes in the doctor - patient relationship and the transformation in the delivery of health care *(A Towle)*.

The following is one example to elucidate the use of the algorithm to choose the most effective line of management as regards (R) iliac fossa pain:

Possible Algorithms:

A.

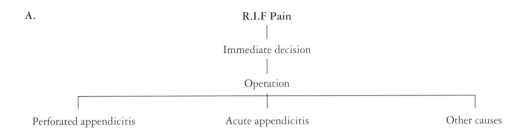

B.

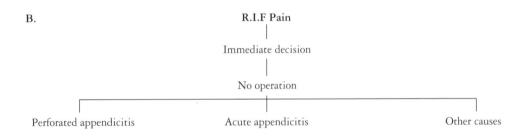

C.

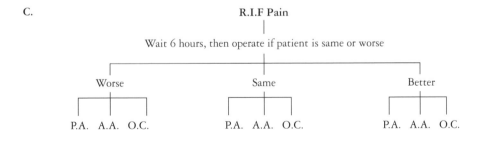

D.

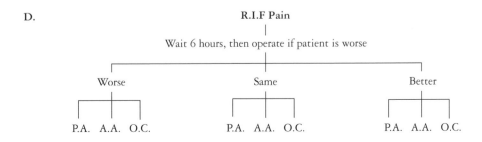

If these four algorithms are evaluated statistically e.g. by using decision trees, one can assess whether the patient ultimately survives or dies as a result of each of these approaches. The endpoint of life or death could, understandably, be considered too drastic and a different endpoint parameter, e.g. length of hospital stay, could be used to evaluate the result of each decision tree. The results will show which algorithms offer the best results, so that success of treatment may be maximised.

Considering the above, one would conclude that the use of Clinical Algorithms should

(i.) be effective education tools,
(ii.) improve patient's care,
(iii.) reduce the cost of care by eliminating use of unnecessary special investigation and other medical technology.

However, scientific evaluation of their effective value in this respect is incomplete.

Limitations of Algorithms

a. Clinical algorithms are best suited for simple problems and it is much more difficult to apply them to complex clinical situations e.g. when patient's complaints cannot fall into one symptom complex. Artificial intelligence will surely help in solving this problem.

b. The clinical algorithm does not consider interaction between factors or variables. Besides this, all variables are always weighted equally.

c. The algorithm may be too deterministic and does not indicate the level of confidence with which the recommendation is made i.e. whether this is a clear-cut decision or a 'close-call'. For this reason, algorithms must be used with good judgement, and one must decide at each step whether the situation in the algorithm still applies to the patient's clinical problem *(Young, M.J., Williams, S.V., Eisenberg, J.M.).*

d. The drawing up of algorithms is influenced by the nature of the clinical judgement of the clinician planning it. Different experts may disagree on the algorithm; i.e. clinical algorithms are as good as the logic of their designer.

Information Technology

It may be concluded from the above, that humans are sub-optimal Bayes Theory and algorithm appliers because different persons use diverse basis for computation. One would think that computerized decision-support systems are the obvious answer, but this is limited by the fact that data used in such systems are themselves subject to human interpretation in the light of human experience and mental models.

There has been an exponential improvement in information technology that includes Internet, the World Wide Web and advances in personal computer systems such as miniaturisation. Palm tops can help in reducing prescribing errors and even provide clinical decision support at a distance from medical centres. Such advances have necessarily had an effect on surgical diagnosis and surgical practice in general, indicating the need for training in Information Technology (IT) of the undergraduate and the poorly IT literate older surgeon. Practically all the new medical graduates are well acquainted with the use of information technology and internet. Tapping into thousands of minds on a particular problem in an online dialogue carries an enormous potential as regards problem solving and decision making. Even conservatively inclined clinicians have been forced to adapt to this because of its many advantages.

As computer hardware becomes cheaper and more powerful, software is becoming a limiting factor in the application of information technology. There are distinct difficulties in commissioning the right systems and one can easily become an object of 'economic blackmail' because it would be too expensive to change a system, in the face of soaring prices and poor service. The adoption of free software, which is licensed by General Public Licence (GPL) allows free downloading from Internet. It is reliable, secure and facilitates the provision of common software components, which can be maintained indefinitely. The adoption of such systems by the E.U. and others has resulted in the availability of high quality programmes worldwide *(Carnall, D.)*.

Information technology is most helpful for patient administration, electronic patient records and more specifically, decision support systems. The latter may help the inexperienced surgeon facing a complex decision, the experienced one to increase the quality of his decision, or the occasional user who requests help in extraordinary cases. Precision, integrity and privacy in the formulation, transmission and collection of such information, e.g. for pathology results and diagnosis, must be assured. To some extent, cryptography may help in this respect. The widespread use of such systems is best controlled by a specialised body, which assures standards in this revolutionary conversion from paperwork to electronics. One advantage of computer-assisted diagnosis is that the operator is forced to be disciplined and precise in his data collection, recording and method. Though this should also apply to the conventional clinical method, there is no such coercion except the dictates of ones self-discipline and conscience. With the more recent technological advances and applications, computer-aided diagnosis has been used in mammography, bone density studies and E.C.G. If such methods are applied to screening programmes, they may ease the manpower requirements. Telemedicine has been used for remote diagnosis, as well as management, in remote areas. It does present a logistic problem, in that it requires the simultaneous presence of busy clinicians at both ends and a good grounding in I.T. communication.

The need for rapid exchange of medical information has become more pressing because of people's increased mobility. Medical information may eventually be made available using a web browser user interface, making sure of security identification and patient consent as part of the access control. One possibility is to use the patient's fingerprints, iris or smart card as an access key, though this is surely nowhere near foolproof *(Balteskard, L., Rinde, E.)*.

Clinical databases are useful in carrying out evaluative research, for clinical audit, for informing management of services, in evaluating outcomes of care, supporting shared decision making models and may help in the planning of medical services. The Directory of Clinical Database *(DoCDat)*, helps in coning down on a particular problem and in indicating suitability and accuracy.

The value of information technology in literature searching (through Medline and the World Wide Web) is only marred by the poor quality control. Internet availability ought to affect research favourably, at least in that one is not forced to resort to industry to pay for access. Electronic publishing is likely to become more popular because of reduced costs and increased accessibility. This increased accessibility is also available to patients and may well result in problems in addition to benefits. The introduction of electronic publishing e.g. netprints, where publishing occurs before peer review, may be regarded as the 'glasnost' of research but will add to the load of external clinical evidence, some of which may be of doubtful value But then, so is a lot of the material that goes through conventional publishing. Regulating the quality of health information on the internet is difficult. Several 'tools' have been suggested for the purpose, but since quality is inherently a subjective assessment, their practical value is limited *(Delamothe)*. Consumers should be instructed how to use this information critically in the same way that we cope with the pervasive advertising that everybody is subjected to.

Information technology has already induced fundamental changes in clinical practice. These changes will surely increase in the future though the implications are not clear. Will these changes result in increased demand due to reduced barriers? How will these demands be filtered? Will productivity improve? How will patients' records be shared? How can one safeguard confidentiality and guard against inappropriate use of patient data? *(Wyatt, J.C., Keen, J.)*. The problems of such innovations can only be unravelled through research and debate by the people involved in their clinical use.

Artificial Neural Networks (ANN)

Artificial Neural Networks models are based on a set of multilayered interconnected equations, which use non-linear statistical analysis to reveal previously unrecognised relations between given input variables and an output variable. In predicting the outcome of acute lower GIT haemorrhage, ANN accuracy varied between 87% and 96% and performed well also in negative prediction, i.e. identifying low risk patients (Das, A. et al.). These models are not meant to replace the experienced clinician but as an aid during triage by ancillary personnel.

Conclusion

Experience, intuition and hard work are still of paramount importance in clinical decision making. Algorithms and other strategies aid but do not replace clinical judgement and their application has recognised limitations.

Chapter 3

Special Investigation

Quotation:

Claude Bernard (1813-1878): 'Man can learn nothing unless he proceeds from the known to the unknown ...... In biological sciences, the role of method is even more important than in the other sciences, because of the complexity of the phenomena and the countless sources of error.'

The immediate and pressing problem posed by the patient is: What must the doctor do, or advise, at that instant? i.e. What is the next step?

Surgical decision making involves three phases i.e. (i) Data Collection, (ii) Data Analysis and (iii) Decision as to patient management. The emphasis is on forming a reasonable working diagnosis and testing it critically rather than wasting everybody's time (including the patient's) collecting superfluous data.

The 'Working Diagnosis' may vary as new clinical data comes in, inducing the clinician to confirm or change his line of management. This might occur at several stages (e.g. in the Out-Patients' or Accident and Emergency Departments), in the ward, once the results of special investigations have been received, in the operating theatre according to operative findings, after receiving the histopathological results, occasionally after passing the test of time, and (hopefully not) after a post-mortem examination (in the latter case the change in management may benefit future patients with similar problems).

Even if one adopts the traditional method of differential diagnosis, provided the various conditions in the list involve the same degree of urgency and do not require any immediate active management, then it is reasonable to request special investigations designed to discriminate between these possibilities, and await results.

Whether one tries to formulate a working diagnosis or a differential diagnosis, detailed history taking and meticulous clinical examinations, with emphasis in the right direction, is fundamental to the proper selection of investigative procedures. Neglect of this principle leads to unnecessary and indiscriminate investigation with its inherent risks, discomfort and expense.

The contemporary faith in science and technology and the belief that the science factor in medicine is increased by the use of technology, has led to a widespread conviction that laboratory results are more accurate, and indeed more helpful than the clinical aspect in surgical management especially if expressed in numbers or graphs, which give an appearance of exactness, but may or may not correspond to the truth (vide Chap 6).

In practice special investigations are useful:

i.   When their results have a direct effect on the decision making in the management pathway or algorithm (e.g. Chart 3.1). There is no justification in endless repetition of tests when normal results are obtained and the patient's clinical condition and therapy remain unchanged. Furthermore, one should avoid attempting to confirm an already proven diagnosis by half-a-dozen different techniques. In short one does the minimum number of investigations that help to resolve the patient's problem e.g. Chart 3.1 and Chart 3.2.

ii. To monitor the course of the disease and/or response to therapy or establish the severity of the disease e.g. U&Es after catheterisation for chronic retention with significant renal impairment; post-operative T-tube Cholangiogram after operative relief of obstructive jaundice; LFTs in cases of jaundice; E.S.R. to monitor the severity of ulcerative colitis and response to therapy; tumour markers after cancer surgery. Even in this respect, experience or experimentation may lead to a conclusion that certain follow-up investigations are not so useful. For example, the benefit of intensive follow-up after surgery for colo-rectal cancer apart from colonoscopy every 2-5 years, has been questioned. One may well agree with this practical view, however, it is useful for the surgeon (if not so much for the patient), to be aware of the rate of his failures.

iii. Uncover or rule out other problems which could affect management.
     The routine ordering of special investigations has been given several labels at various times: 'excessive diagnostic inquisitiveness', 'blunderbuss testing', 'decerebrate medical practice' and 'defensive medicine' (Reiser SJ).
     Factors encouraging the increased use of technology in diagnosis include:
     (i)   The belief by doctors and patients that technology gives more accurate, objective and therefore more scientific data.
     (ii)   Patients are fascinated by the technological aspects of medicine and this attitude is reinforced by the information (or misinformation) in the popular media.
     (iii) The increase in malpractice and compensation suits.
     (iv)   The insurance coverage of medical costs.
     (v)   The increased demand for care due to an aging population.
     (vi)   Guidelines indicating investigations.
     (vii) Higher standards of care.
     (viii) The tendency to make use of a new technology.
     (ix)   The very fact that the tests are available.

Chart 3.1 – *Management of the Clinically Solitary Thyroid Nodule (1987)*

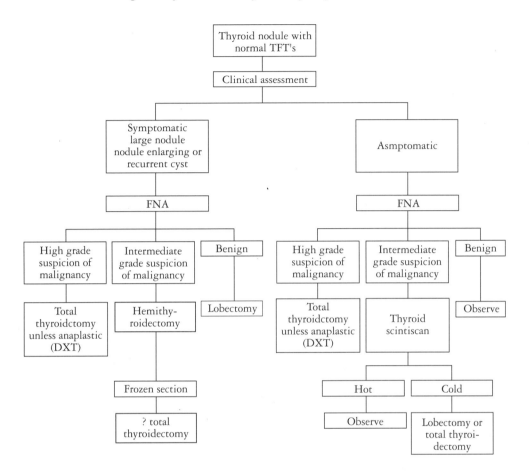

Routine isotope scanning is no longer consedered a mainstay of inverstigation, but may sill be useful as indicated in the above algorithm and when nodularity is associated with hyperthyroidism.

Chart 3.2 – *Investigation of jaundice*

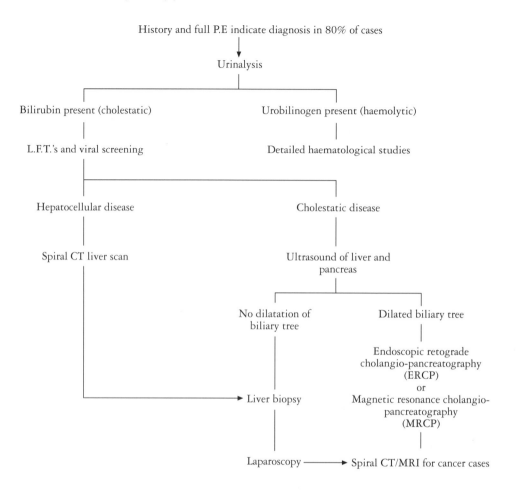

There are also objections levelled at high-tech medicine. Some critics say that considering the demands of other important fields e.g. education and protection of the environment, the state should not spend so much on health. Others say that more emphasis should be placed on preventive medicine. More importantly, it is often pointed out that high technology is often overused and misused. Epidemiologists point out that healthier living owes relatively little to advances in medical technology, but they do not believe that high-tech is dysfunctional in pursuing this goal. This relatively small contribution is well worth pursuing as long as the methods are not misused.

In an effort to encourage more effective use of special investigations, several measures have been used. These include guidelines, the implementation of which involves communication, information and an effort to change attitudes, audit, feedback, peer review and computer reminders. Surprisingly, CME, in its wider sense, does not seem to have the desired effect on the appropriate use of special investigations. One practical measure is to discourage any system whereby doctors get extra remuneration for ordering tests.

Reliance on technologically produced data at the expense of history taking and physical examination is not only wasteful and potentially harmful to the patient, but could lead to (or be the result of) lack of self-confidence by the clinician, reducing his role to that of an intermediary between the patient and the technician. The use of such diagnostic technology could thus be a double-edged sword, helpful when properly used, dangerous for both patient and doctor when misused. The results of special investigations should be seen in their proper perspective: They are not that much more objective than clinical observations since both have to be interpreted by the human mind. Medical technology and its human users are both prone to degrees of variation in accuracy and errors. Fashionable, high-tech investigations are not necessarily more useful than traditional ones: The measurement of invasion depth in melanoma using a ruler is, at present, a much better indicator of prognosis than the expensive use of genetic markers. The best predictors of susceptibility to melanoma are phenotype scales e.g. history of propensity to sunburn, sun exposure, hair colour, number of moles etc. rather than genetic studies or other laboratory tests. Other examples of simple measurements of great practical importance are Apgar scores and Glasgow coma scale *(Rees, J.).* The methodological criteria, by the authors of Standards for Reporting of Diagnostic Accuracy (STARD), should lead to high quality evidence about the usefulness, precision and accuracy of diagnostic tests and the quality of diagnostic articles *(Bussuyt, P.M. et al.).* To properly evaluate the specificity and sensitivity of investigative results, clinicians need to have easy access to this kind of information, delivered in clear and practical language. They have to acquire an acceptable working knowledge of the techniques used. Without this degree of knowledge they cannot subject the evidence from investigations to clinical scrutiny and this may cause regression in intellectual honesty.

Thus the data collected from the steps in the diagnostic process must be adequately sorted out, given their due importance and adequately digested. Whenever possible one correlates the abnormal values of several investigations and a particular disease i.e. a pattern associated with a specific disease or disease complex. Multivariate analysis may be helpful in this respect.

Some special investigations are in themselves invasive and potentially dangerous. The indications for such investigations may be evaluated with the help of decision trees (vide. Chapter on 'Diagnostic Aids'). Ideally the probability of accuracy of any special investigations should be known and the implications of its results weighted accordingly when making a decision. Every item of additional information may constitute a help but may occasionally be a source of confusion. If two tests have a similar value, one should choose the test which will cause the patient the least discomfort. One must keep in mind that each test has a cost in money, danger or discomfort to the patient and in time - in that it may delay a decision in management, if it is superfluous.

Cost-benefit considerations are also important in these days of rationing of health care funding. For example: random colon cancer screening reduces mortality from colon cancer but the cost for each prevented death is considerable. On the other hand selective screening of first and second-degree relatives of patients with colon cancer, especially those with cancer of the colon detected before 45 years of age, carries a distinctly more favourable cost-benefit ratio. Though cost-benefit considerations cannot be ignored when considering the introduction of esoteric technologies, there is sense in making room in the impressive gross expenditure on health for new technologies e.g. CT, MRI, stapling devices, minimal access surgery, etc., which is likely to offer significant improvements in diagnosis and therapy. The most effective ways of maximizing aggregate health gain may, occasionally be unethical: e.g. One can maximize the efficiency of health care by excluding the elderly, cancer cases and other high risk, low salvage cases from such care. This is unacceptable because it implies the subordination of the health needs of the individual to something purely abstract. When resources are limited, as they often are, and priorities have to be set, this is probably best done on the basis of individual need rather than on the basis of aggregate health care of the whole community. This is undoubtedly difficult but not impossible. Though on the surface, this may sound terribly anti-social; the other alternative may heavily favour some sectors and penalize others.

Investigations in Surgical Practice

The aims of diagnostic tests include: detection of disease, supporting clinical management, assessing prognosis, monitoring the clinical course and measuring fitness e.g. for an operative procedure.

In assessing the appropriateness of a diagnostic test to clinical practice the clinician must consider three distinctive points that influence the test's performance:

(i)   the clinical suspicion of the surgeon,
(ii) the clinical condition of the patient,
(iii) the clinical setting in which the test is ordered.

(i)   Clinical Suspicion:
      If the suspicion is strong one needs a test with a high prediction for positive test result, to confirm the diagnosis. For example, if the index of suspicion that a breast lump is malignant, is high, then it is justified to perform a Trucut core biopsy to confirm your working hypothesis. If the clinical suspicion is low, one needs a test with a high prediction for a negative result, to exclude the diagnosis. In this case, if the index of suspicion that the breast lump is

malignant is low, then a Trucut core biopsy may not be the most appropriate investigation, because a 'non-malignant result' could either mean that the lesion is truly benign, or that the sampling was faulty. In such a case, an open biopsy would give a surer reliability for a negative result to exclude the diagnosis of malignancy.

(ii) The Clinical Condition of the Patient:

This may effect the sensitivity or specificity of the test, e.g. patient on oral contraceptives having thyroid function tests may get misleading results. Besides, the patient may be unfit for the diagnostic procedure, or, because of the patient's clinical status, the information gained from the particular investigation would not influence management decisions. More accurate tests may not necessarily effect management. E.g. brain scans in known untreatable neurological conditions.

(iii) The Clinical Setting:

This will influence the clinician's interpretation of a test's usefulness. Specificity and sensitivity of a particular test, whether it is a clinical sign or a special investigation, may change in different settings, e.g. when applied to primary, secondary or tertiary care. If one takes appendicitis as an example of a disease and RIF tenderness as an example of a test, it is reasonable to assume that only patients with doubtful diagnosis who continue to exhibit RIF tenderness are referred further on along the referral pathway. This sample of patients will thus contain an ever-increasing proportion of false positives, the true negatives and obvious true positives having been eliminated along the way. In other words, the easier cases which can be diagnosed with confidence as 'surely appendicitis' or 'surely not appendicitis' are dealt with earlier in the referral pathway by relatively junior clinicians. This leads to a fall in specificity of the test as one moves from the primary to the tertiary care setting. Experimentally specificity has been calculated to fall from 89% in primary care to 16% in tertiary care. In other words, the diagnostic value of RIF tenderness as a test has been used up along the referral pathway *(Sackett, D.L., Haynes, R.B.)*. If a disease occurs uncommonly even tests with high specificity and sensitivity will not have a high accuracy for positive and negative predictions.

It is clear that decisions on management can only be as accurate as the data on which they are based. However, the methodology for assessment of diagnostic techniques is less advanced than that for treatments. The most relevant questions to ask to assess the value of diagnostic tests are: Do test results in affected individuals differ from those in normal individuals? Are patients with abnormal test results more likely to have the target disorder? Do test results distinguish patients with and without the target disorder amongst those suspected of having it? Does the diagnostic test lead to an improvement in outcomes? *(Sackett, D.L., Haynes, R.B.)*.

Investigating Wisely

Before requesting a special investigation one must consider:

(i)   the invasiveness of the procedure,

(ii) the expected information yield,

(iii) the specificity of the investigation - This expresses the proportion of patients without the disease who have a negative test as a factor of 1. The false-positive rate is 1 minus specificity.

(iv) its reliability

(v)   The sensitivity of a test expresses the proportion of patients who have the disease and give a positive result to the test, as a factor of 1 e.g. If free air under the diaphragm in an erect CXR is found in 75% of perforated peptic ulcers the sensitivity of the test is 0.75 i.e. True-positive rate. The sensitivity of a test is high when it is positive in a large number of cases with the targeted condition, but may also be positive in a number of other conditions.

The relative diagnostic accuracy of a test is only clinically important when it is proved to have advantages over a previously used test by a properly conducted study. The discriminatory power (accuracy) of a test is best evaluated by comparing to a gold standard or the closest possible standard test approaching this. However, such reference standards are not always available, and when they are, may have to be changed as a result of new developments *(Knottnerus, J.A., van Weel, C., Muris, J.W.M.)*. The rapidity of development of new diagnostic techniques and technologies, e.g. in imaging, can pose problems, which can be partly overcome by using cross sectional assessment of data on the accuracy of the individual techniques.

From a mathematical point of view the decision to perform an investigation depends on

1. the discriminating power of the test
2. the Prior Probability of the disease which depends on:
   (i)   the prevalence of the disease
   (ii) Clinical and other data indicating the use or otherwise of the test.
3. Patient's utilities or attitude about outcomes.

The most clinically relevant figure is the Post-test probability. This is the proportion of patients with a positive test who actually have the disease. The basis of a probabilistic analysis of information about an investigation is the 2 x 2 Contingency table *(Clarke, C.Z., Hayword, O'Donnell)*.

	D+	D-
T+	TP	FP
T-	FN	TN

D+ = Disease present   TP = True positive
D- = Disease absent   FP = False positive
T+ = Test positive   FN = False negative
T- = Test negative   TN = True Negative

$$\text{Sensitivity} = \frac{TP}{D+} = \frac{TP}{TP + FN} = \text{True positive rate}$$

$$\text{Specificity} = \frac{TN}{D-} = \frac{TN}{TN + FP} = \text{True negative rate}$$

$$\text{False positive rate} = \frac{FP}{D-} = \frac{FP}{TN + FP} = 1\text{- Specificity}$$

$$\text{Prevalence} = \frac{D+}{\text{All patients}} = \frac{D+}{(D+)+(D-)} = \text{Pre test probability or Prior probability}$$

$$\text{Predictive value of a positive test} = \frac{TP}{TP + FP} = \text{Post test probability or posterior probability.}$$

The Odds of an event happening are the probability that it will happen divided by the probability that it will not i.e. $\text{Odds} = \dfrac{P}{1 - P}$

The above-mentioned values related to a particular investigation may be influenced by a number of factors. For example, the false-negative rates for sentinel node biopsy are related to:

1. Quantitative training, i.e. after 30 training operations the FN rate is consistently just less than 10%.
2. The use of both dye and isotopes, i.e. with dye alone a FN rate of 33% was obtained.
3. Timing of isotope and dye injection. The best results were obtained when the dye was injected between 5 and 30 minutes before operation and the isotope on the same day of operation.
4. Site of injection of dye and isotope. Intra-tumour injection seems to give the best results for para-sternal nodes.
5. Multi-focal tumours are associated with a higher FN rate.
6. A high S-rate fraction, i.e. the DNA synthesis phase when the cancer cells are not dividing in a higher proportion of cases *(Bergkvist, L., et al.)*.

Sensitivity and specificity can be more easily understood using visual aids (Loong T-W):

Symbols used for visual aids

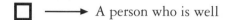 A person who is well

A person who has disease

A negative result

A positive result

A well person who tests negative (T.N.)

A diseased person who tests positive (T.P.)

A well person who tests positive (F.P.)

A diseased person who tests negative (F.N.)

Sensitivity: *refers to how good a test is at correctly identifying people who have the disease*

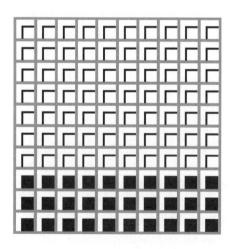

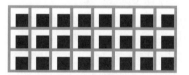

Sensitivity is 24/30=80%

Results of a diagnostic test on a hypothetical population of a 100

Specificity: *Refers to how good a test is at identifying people who are well*

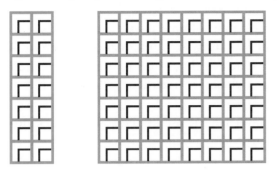

Specificity = 56/70 = 80%

Positive Predictive Value: *refers to the chance that a positive test result is correct.*

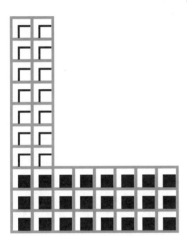

Positive Predictive Value = 24/63 = 63%

Negative Predictive Value: *refers to the chance that a negative result is correct*

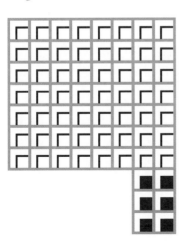

Negative Predictive Value = 56/62 = 90%

Hypothetical population

As the prevalence of a disease decreases, the Positive Predictive Value will fall, while the Negative Predictive Value will increase.

Computer analysis may help by measuring the information yield of each test and perhaps incorporating into the decision making system information on the cost-benefit balance for each investigation. One can thus optimise the investigation plan, reducing the use of investigations, which are hazardous, uncomfortable or have a low information yield.

In the absence of computer aids the clinician must take the above factors into consideration when he draws his investigation plan. The science of making best use of data is what the surgeon should strive to perfect during his training and throughout his life. It is obvious, however, that there is a need for formal standards governing the acceptance of new diagnostic techniques in clinical practice. Agreement on these formal standards is not easy because of difficulties such as operator dependence, quantification of vague outcomes e.g. pain, confidence with the technique an d instrumental variation.

Special Investigation Modes

Special investigations are a means of obtaining useful information on the state of the patient. This may be considered in one of three modes:

1. Static - they pinpoint the anatomic condition or biochemical status at any given instant,
2. Dynamic - one measures the rate of anatomical or physiological changes e.g. tests measuring rates of blood flow, rates of pulmonary gas exchange, ECG, EEG, changes in the results of static investigations performed serially.
3. Imaging.

See Chart 3.3.

It is not irrelevant to insist at this stage on what may, perhaps, be considered commonplace: Writing on the request form should be legible.

Chart 3.3 – *Classification of Special Investigations*

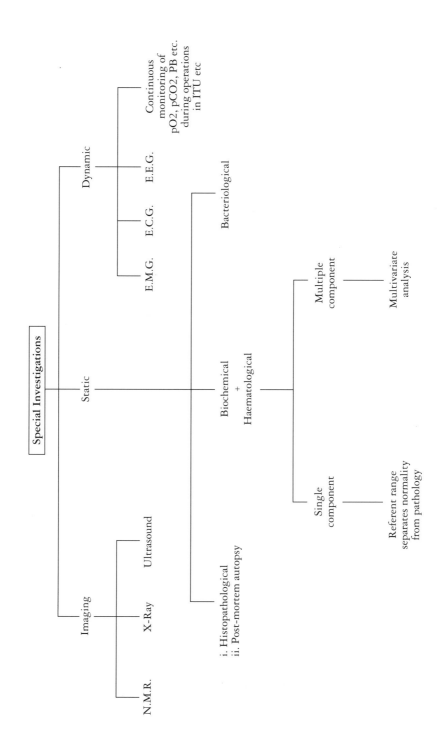

The patient's particulars, ward designation, the Consultant's name, the date, the Hospital 'unit' number, results of similar previous (or other relevant) tests with dates, relevant drug therapy, as well as the investigation requested should be clearly written. We must help our colleagues in the lab, that they may help us and our patients.

The clinician should bear clearly in mind that it is the result of the investigation that is important, not the dispatch of the specimen. When a patient's life depends on getting a result rapidly, then not only may the housemen have to take the specimen to the laboratory, but he may have to call back in person or telephone to get the result quickly.

Biochemical and Haematological Investigations

To obtain static biochemical and haematological information, several technologies are applied including spectrophotometry, fluorometry, potentiometry, scintillation counting, chromatography, electrophoresis, as well as specific enzymatic and immunological techniques.

Dynamic tests are conceivable in the biochemical field by monitoring rapid changes in concentration of metabolites using the same techniques as in getting static biochemical information. With modern technology these assessments can be performed in real time e.g. assessments of pO_2 and pCO_2 during operations, in H.D.U. and in I.T.U.

Though automated technology can carry out more tests at lower cost, this has led to routine packaging of results instead of a specific single test which one may need. This, in fact, increases the number of laboratory tests performed not necessarily with a corresponding increase in benefit.

Tumour Markers

These are substances associated with the presence and growth of tumours.

Ideally, a tumour marker is detectable in the patient's blood, is tumour specific, organ specific and perhaps, proportional to tumour mass. In fact, present tumour markers do not satisfy all these criteria e.g. CEA and PSA (20% of men with prostatic cancer have normal PSA values; whilst 25% of men with BPH have high PSA levels, i.e. Specificity and sensitivity are far from ideal). A tumour marker can be detected in a solid tumour, in circulating tumour cells in the peripheral blood, in lymph nodes, in bone marrow, or in other body fluids e.g. urine or stools.

The main uses of tumour markers are:
(i)   Screening for primary disease
(ii)   Diagnosis of primary disease e.g. the presence of fusion protein PAYS-PPAR is found only in thyroid follicular carcinoma cells and can help to distinguish thyroid follicular carcinoma and follicular adenoma.
(iii) Monitoring treatment
(iv)   Follow-up to detect recurrences.

(v) Therapy options e.g.(oestrogen receptors).

(vi) Staging e.g. regional lymph node CEA estimations during colon cancer surgery. The techniques used so far are of the static investigation type. This may involve estimation of monoclonal antibodies, immunohistochemistry, reversed transcriptase and polymerase chain reaction. In general, tumour markers may be secreted into the blood, expressed on the cell surface and thus measurable only from biopsy specimens, or expressed as genomic sequences which indicate an increased susceptibility (rather than a certainty) to develop a particular malignancy.

Examples of presently used tumour markers fall into three categories:

1. Secretion of products or enzymes – e.g. S. alkaline phosphatase in bone or liver secondaries. These can then be differentiated by estimating isoenzymes. Also 5-HIAA in carcinoid syndrome, Alpha-foeto protein in hepatocellular carcinoma and PSA in carcinoma of the prostate.

2. Structural molecules – e.g. CEA in colorectal cancer as well as in regional lymph nodes of colonic malignancy and CA 125 in ovarian cancer.

3. Products of cell turnover or proliferation – e.g. Lactate dehydrogenase levels in Seminomas (non-specific) *(Hanning, I., Dow, E.).*

Specificity in tumour markers refers to:

(i) Tumour specific proteins- a fusion protein associated with a malignant process in which an oncogene is translocated and fused to an active promoter of another gene.

(ii) Cell specific proteins overexpressed in malignant cells- i.e. proteins expressed normally in differentiated cells, but at higher rates in corresponding tumour cells e.g. P.S.A., tyrosinase protein in melanocytes.

(iii) Non-specific proteins e.g.Oncofetal antigens, such as CEA and Alphafetoprotein in hepatocellular tumours but also in testicular and ovarian cancer *(Lindblom, A., Liljegren, A.).*

There are general considerations, which require emphasis:

(i)   No serum marker in current use is specific for malignancy.

(ii)   Early malignancy is rarely associated with elevated tumour marker levels.

(iii) High levels are usually associated with advanced disease.

(iv)   Absolute organ specificity has not been attained. One of the best performers is PSA, which is only relatively organ specific.

(v)   No tumour marker is elevated in 100% of cases with a particular malignancy with the exception of HCG in choriocarcinoma.

(vi)   In the diagnosis of an unknown primary, requesting a range of tumour markers is not useful.

(vii) Reference ranges of tumour markers are only for guidance. Variation in levels over a period of time are more relevant.

(viii) Results of tumour marker assays are specific to the type of kit and method used and this should be indicated in the report.

The following is a list of sensitivity and specificity of commonly used tumour markers:

Marker	Cancer	Sensitivity	Specificity
AFP	Hepatocellular	98%	65%
CA 19.9	Pancreatic	78-90%	95%
CA 27.29	Breast	62%	83%
CA 15.3	Ovarian	46%	99%
CA 125	Colorectal	40-47%	90%
	Breast	45%	81%
	Recurrent disease	84%	100%
HCG	Trophoblastic	100%	100%
PSA	Prostatic	57-93%	55-68%
	w/age-specific range	95%	88%
	W/8 micro g/L cutoff and exclude BPH, advanced prostate Ca.		
CA 72-4	Gastric	62.5%	90%
CA 19-9	Pancreatic	57%	90%
TK	Melanomas; Sarcomas	53%	90%
			(Kausitz, J., Pecen, L.)

TMUGS

This stands for Tumour Marker Utility Grading System (American Society of Clinical Oncology). The scoring is from 0 to 3+, basing on levels of evidence, with 0 meaning the test is of no utility and 3+ meaning it is very valuable, with gradations in between. Most tumour markers fall in the low level of evidence categories.

Genomic Investigations and Genetic Research

Genetically determined diseases include those resulting from:

(a) Chromosomal abnormalities e.g. Down's, Klinefelter's and Turner's syndromes.

(b) Single gene disorders e.g. Familial polyposis coli, neurofibromatosis and achondroplasia.

(c) Unusual patterns of inheritance (Trinucleotide repeat expansion mutations) e.g.

Myotonic dystrophy.

(d) Interaction of genetic and environmental factors e.g. Arteriosclerosis and neural tube defects.

The concept of the genome as representing a blueprint of human nature is not an absolute novelty. It closely resembles the Aristotelian idea of 'eidos' and Thomas Aquinas' notion of 'forma' or 'soul'. The genome is seen as the core of our nature and synonymous with personal identity. This notion is not completely acceptable if one considers the situations that occur in monozygotic twins and cloning where the genes are identical but the persons unquestionably distinct *(Mauron, A.)*. The term 'genome' here refers to the totality of a species' genes, or DNA sequences.

Genomic research and investigations has to be viewed in its proper perspective. They may be useful in:

(i)   Identifying individual predisposition to disease e.g. Factor V Leiden as a risk factor for thromboembolism.

(ii)   Creating new categories of special investigations.

(iii)   Measuring responsiveness to drugs.

(iv)   Measuring possibility of adverse drug reactions. The latter two applications are influenced by behavioural and environmental factors in addition to genetic ones.

(v)   Diagnosis of pathogens.

(vi)   Diagnosis or staging of disease with new diagnostic and prognostic markers.

(vii)   Close reading of the human genome will help our understanding of human variation in health and disease, linking clinical heterogenicity to biological diversity and correlating genomic findings to clinical outcome. Using the usual histological and immunohistochemical methods, it may be difficult or impossible to draw sharp boundaries between different types or subtypes of certain tumours e.g. soft tissue tumours, and this leads to uncertainty in diagnosis. Genome-wide analysis helps in drawing up these boundaries and thus in the differential diagnosis. These investigations also distinguish subtypes, explaining and predicting their different natural history and clinical behaviour.

(viii) Creating new therapeutic targets.

Potential practical applications:

1. Monogenic diseases – About 5000 diseases are inherited in Mendelian fashion, but these are quite rare e.g. inborn errors of metabolism, inherited haemoglobinopathies, cystic fibrosis and haemophilia. The global prevalence of all single gene disorders is about 1%.

2. Infectious diseases – Knowledge of mechanisms of viral action at molecular level has led to the development of antiviral therapies. Other applications include:

the understanding of mechanisms of virulence in bacteria, the development of diagnostic agents, development of vaccines e.g. against Neisseria meningitidis, study of population genetics, dynamics and ecology of infectious diseases e.g. virulent forms of E. coli causing food poisoning and variant Creuzfeldt – Jacob disease. Genomics are also useful in vector control e.g. using transposons to alter mosquito genomes, as well as understanding the variability of host response e.g. to malaria.

3. Cancer – Many cancers require the acquisition of multiple oncogenes mutation. Different patterns of gene expression carry different prognoses e.g. in breast cancer. One expects genomic research will result in a more scientific approach to classification and therapy. In familial neoplasms, e.g. retinoblastoma, familial polyposis coli, genomic investigation allows exclusion from opportunistic screening of cases of cases who do not carry the suppressor gene mutation. It is still premature however, to use genomic techniques in public health programmes for the prevention of cancer.

4. Complex multifactorial diseases – Genomics help in identifying the different genes involved in the variable susceptibility to environmental agents or the effects of aging. This may lead to more focussed public health measures and targeted therapy e.g. diabetes, myocardial ischaemia and asthma.

5. Developmental defects and mental retardation – genomics allow a more precise analysis of chromosomal abnormalities as a basis for developmental defects e.g. skeletal malfomations.

6. Ageing – provides new insights into the biology of aging and age-related diseases.

7. Therapy – It allows individualised tailoring of drug therapy through the identification of polymorphisms in metabolic pathways.

8. Gene therapy – refers to the treatment of disease by altering the genetic make-up of cells, organs or individuals. This may take the form of: (i) Germ-line gene therapy, which involves the introduction of foreign DNA into the fertilized egg. This is banned in most countries. (ii) Somatic cell gene therapy where the genome of cells of individual organs or tissues is altered. These alterations are not passed to the offspring. This technique has not been very successful so far.

9. Stem cell therapy – This technique is still in its early stages. It involves the treatment of the nuclei of adult cells so that they can be induced to differentiate into specific tissue types for therapeutic purposes i.e. therapeutic cloning or the use of embyonic stem cells

10. Plant genomics – intended to increase resistance to pathogens or to increase the crop's nutritional content, in the fight against hunger. The same technique is used in the production of edible vaccines e.g. Hepatitis B and cholera.

11. Forensic medicine – for DNA 'fingerprinting'.

12. Biotechnology – e.g. for the production of diagnostic agents and kits.

These new developments may change the emphasis from one concentrated on existing disease to one mainly directed towards prediction and prevention. They may result in the development of new therapeutic and immunization targets and drastic changes in medical education.

As with all new technologies one has to be aware of the potential risks:

(i)   Attempts to help individuals and families with genetic diseases may result in increase in the number of defective genes in the human gene pool.

(ii) To date, the risk benefit ratio of germ-line gene therapy is unfavourable. Unpredictable effect may be passed on to offspring.

(iii) Possibilities of misuse of genetic databases by insurance companies, government bodies, the legal profession, police or individuals.

(iv) Commercial ownership may lead to ethical and economic problems.

(v)   These technologies may be applied to biological warfare and other political misuse.

Confirmation of a diagnosis in some diseases involves biopsy and histopathological results. Since the histological picture is an expression of the genetics, one may conceive that genomic based diagnosis e.g. by DNA microarray, should constitute a major breakthrough. Such special investigations are certainly helpful for identifying disease subtypes and therefore helping to understand the wide variation in outcome of certain diseases (See table below). It should also help in fine-tuning of diagnostic resolution and may provide prognostic indications. As indicated in the above list of uses, results of genomic investigations may correlate with clinical outcome e.g. in B-cell lymphomas, melanomas and breast carcinomas. These techniques may also prove helpful in non-malignant diseases, especially those associated with low diagnostic resolution e.g. auto-immune disorders *(Brugarolas, J., Haynes, B.F., Nevins, J.R.)*.

The sequencing and analysis of the human genome may well lead to the discovery of the underlying mechanisms of disease. This would enable us to ration diagnostic and therapeutic methods targeting these mechanisms; e.g. In a biopsy specimen of a malignant tumour, one could find that the DNA repair genes are turned off, which would indicate that radiotherapy is likely to be beneficial. During opportunistic screening of members of a family where cases of Familial polyposis coli have occurred, the absence of the corresponding gene can avoid the discomfort, dangers and expense of repeated endoscopic investigations.

These potential applications of genetics to clinical medicine have generated a lot of excitement. One must, however, sort out the hypothesis from the hype, not overestimating the potential of genomic research. The genome provides description of genes but gives no indication as to function. Besides, the complement of human genes is much smaller than previously thought. Of the 26000 to 38000 genes in the human genome, only about 900 are linked to disease and most are rare single-gene diseases. Even amongst these, there are single-gene disorders with a high

Disease	Subtype	Correlation	*Reference*
Beta cell lymphoma	(a) Germinal centre type accoding to pattern of gene expression	76%-5years survival	*(Alizadeh, A.A., Eisen, M.P. et al.)*
	(b) Mature activated type	16% 5-years survival	
Carcinoma of the breast	(a) Oestrogn receptor+ve	i. Correlation with Erb 2	*(Perou, C.M., Serlie, T., Eisen, M.P. et al.)*
	(b) Oestrogen receptor-ve	ii.Correlation with tumours resembling basal cell carcinomas	
Melanomas	(a) Less aggressive cluster	Correlates with in vitro behavior. Unproved clinical correlation	*(Bitter, M., Meltzer, P., Chen, Y.)*
	(B)More aggressive	Correlates with in vitro behaviour. Unproved clinical correlation.	

predictive value, e.g. the gene for Huntington's disease and there are others, which carry a low predictive value because of the influence of other genes and environmental factors. Our knowledge of genes linked with more common complex-trait diseases is in its infancy, with poor understanding of the significance of genomic sequencing. These diseases develop because of the interaction of several genes with low penetrance, environmental factors and behaviour, e.g. heart disease, asthma, diabetes mellitus etc. Genetic investigations have low predictive value in such cases. One has to remember that inherited forms of cancer represent only about 5% of adult cancer. Even when a particular disease is inherited as an autosomal dominant, there is only a 50 – 50 chance of inheriting it *(Weitzel, J.N., McCahill, L.E.)*. In those that carry the susceptibility gene, the risks and benefits of prophylactic surgery must be balanced against the efficacy of screening and the risks of the disease itself. Phenotype of disease does not necessarily reflect genotype, because of the influence of environment and behaviour. Investigating such interactions is a challenge which may prove difficult to tackle as well as expensive. Anthony, Eaton and Henderson, in 1995, coined the term 'envirome' referring to the totality of environmental influences. Conclusions linking genes to disease require confirmation by epidemiological studies *(Senior, K.)*.

This rapid development of genomic technology will surely have an impact on several aspects of medical practice: there must be adequate regulation of its funding, research practice and application as well as the confidentiality of data and results.

Results of genetic investigation could have a clear impact on insurance aspects and on employment. Involvement of the private sector in a big way could have both positive and negative effects, which will be referred to shortly. Health Services have to train their staff so that they can collaborate with and correctly use, the genetic service. An administrative framework has to be created for an expanding genetic service and for opportunistic screening *(Zimmerman, R., Emery, J., Richards, T.)*. It is necessary to educate both the public and the policy-makers as to the implications of genomics and the related technology. Finally this enthusiasm concentrated on the potential of genomic research should not distract us from tackling the more tangible environmental and social issues.

The Relationship between Genetic and Environmental Factors

Quantitative genetic research designs generally follow any of three avenues: family, twin and adoption studies, each having its advantages and disadvantages. From such studies it is clear that genes are not all-important. Environment and chance events may also shape outcomes. Genes are regulated by promoter genes which can be turned on and off by environmental factors. Thus, genes are enablers and not constrainers! When conducting genetic molecular studies, one uses allelic association and linkage analysis. The genome and the envirome operate together by correlation and interaction. Furthermore, correlation may be passive, evocative or active. Passive correlation is most important in infancy and early childhood when parents are the main environmental influences. Thus the entire child's genome and partly his early envirome depend on the parents' genotype. Evocative correlation occurs when the child starts to evoke responses from a wider social environment. Active correlation occurs when one actively tries to find an environment that is congenial to one's genetic constitution. Genotype-environment interaction addresses the various degrees by which either of these two factors, separately or together, influence the phenotype, either in a positive or in a negative (i.e. protective) manner. Thus the combination of molecular genetic techniques with genotype-environment correlation and interaction, allows specific genes to be associated with specific environments, offering an insight into these mechanisms *(Neiderhiser, J.M.)*. Genetic mutations may cause complex diseases and affect response to therapy.

Single Nucleotide Pleomorphism (SNP) is an inherited DNA sequence variation occurring in 1 in 1000 to 2000 nucleotide bases, producing human genetic variation. 1.42 million of these have been found in the human genome, indicating a considerable variation in the latter *(Editorial: The Lancet .Vol.357 2001)*.

The identification of highly penetrant, susceptibility-conferring, genotypes, or those indicating inherited drug susceptibility, are important and will surely become more so in the future. These categories, however, do not represent such a large proportion of the population that would warrant a general screening programme *(Holtzman, N.A. et al.)*. One can refer to the list of criteria for screening programmes further on in this chapter. Perhaps, opportunistic screening of persons with a relevant family history would be more reasonable.

Most of the major risk factors to human disease e.g. malnutrition, poor sanitation, tobacco, alcohol, pollution, trauma etc. are not affected by genetic research or influenced by genomic investigations. Their control and prevention falls in the realm of politics rather than medicine. In fact social, environmental and behavioural factors account for a much larger proportion of disease than genetics. A study involving 90,000 almost-identical and non-identical twins, found that genetic factors have only a minor role in causing cancer of the prostate, large bowel and breast. Environmental factors were major aetiological contributors to cancer in all of the 28 anatomical sites studied *(Lichtenstein, P. et al.)*.The advances in genetics would have more impact if one could determine the genotypes of the majority of people who are likely to suffer from common diseases. The complexity of genetics in such diseases is, however, often quite vast, rendering widespread application of these methods impractical in the near future. On the other hand, the very rarity of a gene defect could suggest how vital that gene is. For example an abnormal transcription factor GATA 3 may produce several defects e.g. deafness, hypoparathyroidism and renal dysplasia *(Barbour, V., Horton, R.)*. The problem is rendered more complex by the fact that the same pathology can result from different combinations of genetic, environmental and behavioural factors. It is becoming increasingly clear that research in clinical medicine, statistics, epidemiology and genetics must interact in order to maximise results.

There is one sobering thought in the midst of this intellectual excitement: Through the exasperation of profits and medicalization (Illich I), the results of genetic research may well be out of the economic reach for a large proportion of the world population.

Molecular Cytogenetics
These techniques may be of diagnostic and prognostic importance in neoplastic conditions. Chromosome abnormalities are either balanced i.e. without visible gain or loss of chromosome material, or unbalanced, with gain or loss of chromosome material e.g. the Philadelphia chromosome in chronic myeloid leukaemia. Conventional banding, and the newer hybridisation techniques are useful in their detection.

Clinical Bacteriology
Infection accounts for about 30% of adult outpatient referrals and approximately 50% of paediatric referrals *(Gorbach, S.L., Mensa, J., Gatell, J.M.)*. Clinical bacteriology is the study of specimens taken from patients suspected of suffering from infectious diseases to find:

(i) whether there is a change in the kind or distribution of normal flora,

(ii) whether potentially pathogenic organisms are the cause of the disease.

These may involve (a) various types of direct microscopy, e.g. in malaria and leprosy,

(b) isolation and identification of the aetiological agent, e.g. in typhoid, infected wound cultures and sensitivity testing etc.

(c) serological techniques for detection of antibody or less commonly specific antigen, e.g. antibody in syphilis and Legionnaire's disease or antigen in diagnosis of hepatitis A, B,C, D and E.

Isolation and identification are the most precise of the three methods mentioned and they provide the only method of getting in vitro sensitivity. However the necessity for speed in reporting the possible pathogen may induce the clinical bacteriologist to issue a series of preliminary reports based on colonial and microscopic morphology e.g. Gram stain in suspected Clostridial infections and other evidence, e.g. growth requirements. In this respect, adequate information regarding the clinical features is invaluable data for the clinical bacteriologist.

New diagnostic techniques are finding a place in the microbiologist's armamentarium. The impetus for new techniques comes from three sources:

(i) The need for more rapid diagnosis of infections caused by micro-organisms that are slow or difficult to grow e.g. mycobacteria.

(ii) To detect low pathogen numbers.

(iii) Discovery of new pathogens or re-emergence of importance of known ones. Molecular diagnostic techniques are examples of this and are slowly gaining acceptance, though there are still problems with methodology, standardization, sensitivity, specificity and cost *(Wilcox, M.H., Warren, N.F.)* .

The role of the clinical bacteriologist has now evolved in such a way that besides assuring that laboratory investigations are carried out as efficiently and economically as possible, he must also collaborate closely with the clinicians. The clinical bacteriologist has become an integral and essential part of a multidisciplinary team, which can then tackle clinical and academic situations more efficiently, for example:

1. In unusual, severe or life-threatening infections that pose diagnostic and/or chemotherapeutic problems.

2. To suggest possible aetiological agents of infection and probable sensitivity patterns when the infecting organisms have not yet been isolated or the relevant specimens were not taken.

3. For fine-tuning of chemotherapeutic strategies to obtain valuable synergic or additive effects.

4. To help in the interpretation of laboratory results e.g. serological tests, direct gram stains, isolation of exotic organisms etc.

5. To advise on preventive measures, chemoprophylaxis and infection control measures.

6. To investigate and publish jointly in peer-reviewed scientific journals new observations or unusual case studies, involving bacteriology, encountered in the course of one's work.

7. To issue and discuss preliminary reports on cases which involve slow growing pathogens.

8. To advise on the proper collection, minimal necessary volume, storage and delivery of specimens to the laboratory.

9. To provide information of epidemiological importance e.g. unusually virulent strains of strep. Pyogenes, E coli 0157 isolates and nosocomial multi-drug resistant pathogens.

10. To introduce and explain current nomenclature and other aspects of taxonomy.

11. To provide an efficient on-call service after normal working hours.

12. To help clinicians decide on the relevance of laboratory findings, especially in the immunocompromised patient, in the light of the clinical information and / or recent surgical interventions.

13. Suggesting optimum lines of investigation and ensure that the efforts of the lab are used to the best advantage *(Cuschieri, P.)*.

The corollary is that the above is an excellent indicator of how a clinician can make best use of a microbiologist's services.

Radiological Investigations

To obtain morphological information, one selects a measurable physical probe - light, sound, X-Rays, NMR - that is effected by a certain property of tissue - its density, elemental composition, elasticity, viscosity, temperature or the electronic structure of individual materials, and uses the appropriate technique to detect and display the image.

One can do this using the naked eye, but often one resorts to technological aids:

(a) **Light-** the laboratory microscope, endoscopes, thermography

(b) **Sound-** ultrasonic reflective imaging has been made possible by accurate measurement of time intervals (originally for radar and sonar). It monitors the reflections from interfaces between tissues. The effectiveness of the reflection depends on the differences in density and speed of sound in different tissues. Doppler techniques measure the velocity of moving objects e.g. RBCs.

(c) **X-Ray-** this is really energetic electromagnetic radiation which is more penetrating than light. Its application distinguishes differences between tissue densities.

(d) **NMR-** images are obtained depending on the hydrogen content and viscosity of tissues and organs. It requires highly sensitive radio frequency technology, the development of large superconductive magnets and computerised image reconstruction.

Endoscopy

This is the process of inspecting both internal body cavities and lumens of epithelial lined organs using rigid or flexible instruments (Plate 4). It is an extension of what is visible to the eye in the clinical examination. Endoscopy may be both diagnostic and therapeutic e.g. polypectomy at colonoscopy, banding of oesophageal varices at OGD and various other types of minimally invasive surgical procedures. The flexible endoscopes use fibreoptics usually combined with a chip camera at the tip of the instrument. Such instruments are used in upper gastro intestinal endoscopy, ERCP, lower gastrointestinal endoscopy, enteroscopy, laparoscopy, bronchoscopy, thoracoscopy, mediastinoscopy, cystoscopy, ureterocopy, arthroscopy, choledochoscopy and brain endoscopy.

At enteroscopy, a special long endoscope is passed beyond the duodenum. These enable visualisation and biopsy of 50% or more of the small bowel. This is not a widely used technique but may be useful in obscure GIT bleeding and in the diagnosis of small bowel tumours (Wilmer, A., Rutgeerts, P.). 'Mother and baby' scopes are so called because one inserts a second thin scope through the biopsy channel. One can use this method to dilate bile duct strictures. This technque does not replace surgical repair but may serve as a temporary measure pre-operatively, if the patient has advanced liver dysfunction, if the patient is unfit for operation and in strictures which are difficult to repair by open surgical methods.

Recent advances in miniaturization and nano technology has enabled the development of pill-like gadgets for endoscopy and chemical investigation of the GIT, which technology will surely be extended to the investigation of other systems. The endoscopic pill, laboratory in a pill and microrobots are under trial. The former two devices are not steerable and rely on peristalsis for their propulsion. The microrobot is semi-autonomous and is capable of an inchworm locomotion system based on vacuum and pressure. It is equipped with a microcamera and the device can be used for colonoscopy, or when swallowed, for whole gut investigation, where it can be made to stop at critical points for more detailed visualisation (*Bradbury, J.*). Their more advanced successors will surely take much of the unpleasantness out of endoscopy as practiced at present.

Oesophageal Manometry and pH

Measuring gastro-oesophageal motility and acid reflux are important adjuncts to endoscopy and radiology and can be performed in an out-patient clinical setting. A special nasogastric tube is passed into the oesophagus in the usual manner. pH and

Plate 4

...inspecting body cavities and lumens...

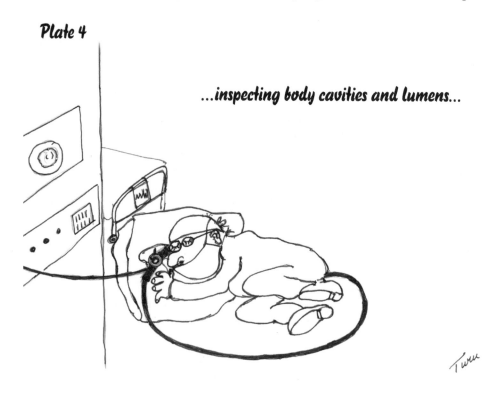

pressure measurements are recorded using a transducer and appropriate recording apparatus. One can distinguish thereby between oesophageal motility problems and reflux.

Radiology

An X-Ray picture depends on four basic densities: a. Air
b. Fat
c. Soft tissues (water density)
d. Calcific

For a structure to cast a discrete shadow it must consist of one of these densities. When requesting a radiograph, or interpreting it, the clinician must rethink the anatomy in terms of the four basic densities described above, and the interfaces they create e.g. it is possible to visualise the size of a kidney in a plain radiograph because it is surrounded by fat.

For the same reason many organs do not cast a discrete shadow but the introduction of a contrast medium might then make it visible, e.g. Barium in the stomach or a water-soluble iodine containing contrast medium in arteries and veins. Negative contrast media, e.g. air or CO_2 are sometimes useful in creating a new interface e.g. double contrast Barium enemata.

The problem of observer variation is very real, as has been shown in many studies *(Burkelo, C.), (Henry Garland, L.), (Tuddenham, W.J.).* This has to be kept in mind when evaluating all clinical evidence. Attributing a mistake to operator dependence of a particular radiological technique (what isn't operator dependent?) does not help one's misdiagnosed patient. It is a pity that radiologists hardly ever attend a ward round, an operative procedure or a post-mortem on patients who required their services. Radiological conferences are helpful but are not enough.

If the above facts are kept in mind, then it will be easier for the clinician to request the appropriate 'basic' radiological investigation.

The rapidity with which technical advances have developed, and the promise of continuing progress, has modified the traditional relationship between the referring clinician and the medical imaging specialist (the new term for the poor old Consultant Radiologist). Difficulties arise in seeking the appropriate use of the facilities. The choice of the imaging technology must take into account the clinical benefit, therapeutic gain, cost and the locally available expertise with the various technologies.

In the past decade and a half, we have had the development of Digital Radiography, Ultrasound Techniques, Nuclear Medicine, Positron Emission Tomography and Nuclear Magnetic Resonance technology in grey scale and colour. Some aspects of these techniques have made the improvements in Interventional Radiology possible.

The following tables show the advantages and disadvantages of each of these investigative procedures:

Conventional CT Scanning

Advantages	Disadvantages
Density differences as small as 0.5% may be differentiated.	Fairly expensive.
It is quantitative (size, density).	Thin patient have poorer resolution for some organs
It is non-invasive, safe and is suitable for out-patient use.	Bone may create some artefacts.
Smaller and deeper lesions can be detected compared to conventional radiography and radionuclide scans.	Frequently requires use of I.V. contrast with potential allergic manifestations.
Allows assessment of soft tissues in contrast to conventional X-ray technology.	Prone to artefacts from movement and breathing.
Serves as a guide for interventional techniques.	Scan time is slow.
Main role is now in non-contrast exams that do not require fast scanning e.g. cerebral infarcts and haemorrhage.	Difficult to reformat in different planes.
	Dynamic contrast studies not possible.
	Small lesions between slices may be missed.

Figure 3.1 – *Advantages and disadvantages of Conventional CT Scanning (Crockford, M.)*

Spiral CT Scanner

A single X-Ray beam rotates round patient while the latter is moved in the axis, producing a spiral course of the beam.

Advantages	Disadvantages
Scan time is much shorter than conventional CT.	Slower than a multislice scanner.
Thin slices even in different planes are possible.	
Dynamic contrast studies and even angiographic work, in different phases of contrast enhancement, are possible.	
Less likely to miss small lesions.	
Enables interventional procedures in real time.	
Cheaper than a multislice scanner.	

Figure. 3.2 – *Advantages and disadvantages of the Spiral CT Scanner. (Garvey, C.J., Hanlon, R.)*

Multislice Scanner

Multiple detectors (up to 8) rotate in a spiral round patient.

Advantages	Disadvantages
Faster then spiral scanner.	More expensive to buy.
Better patient throughput.	More expensive maintenance.
Better for uncooperative, dyspnoeic or trauma patients.	More time necessary to analyse data.
Larger area covered during a single acquisition.	Increased radiological workload.
Less movement artefact.	Higher radiation dose than spiral CT.
Lifelike multiplanar reformats.	
Improved cardiac and vascular imaging.	

Figure. 3.3 *Advantages and disadvantages of the Multislice CT Scanner (Garvey, C.J., Hanlon, R.).*

Positron Emission Tomography

The technique is based on the detection of radioactivity emitted after a small amount of radioactive tracer is injected into a peripheral vein. The positrons emitted collide with electrons in the tissues, emitting photons. These are detected by scintillation crystals placed round the patient which convert them first to light and then electrical signals.

Advantages	Disadvantages
There is a choice of chemical elements of labelling e.g. (O_2, N_2, C_{11}, N_{13} F-fluorodeoxyglucose) each with a very short half-life.	The radionuclides have a very short half-life and so must be made close to the point of detection.
Physiological processes can be measured.	Only biochemical processes with fast rates of turnover can be measured.
Tissue injury can be detected very early.	Expensive and requires high technology.
High sensitivity.	The resolution is only 5mm in exposures of 1 minute.
May help to distinguish between benign and malignant tumours by measuring the rate of consumption of glucose; investigating strokes and dementia, assessing viable myocardium and distinguishing between recurrent tumour and radiation necrosis by measuring oxygen consumption.	Low specificity. e.g. Trauma vs infection vs tumour hardly distinguishable.

Figure 3.4 *– Advantages and disadvantages of Positron Emission Tomography.*

F-fluorodeoxyglucose (F.D.G.) is an analogue of glucose and mimics its cellular uptake and initial metabolism enabling cells using excess glucose to be visualised. This increased glucose metabolism is most commonly seen in malignant tissues and some benign disorders. The main application of PET has been in lung tumours, including their more accurate staging and semi-qualitative analysis, which are prognostically significant, colorectal cancers, especially recurrent disease and hepatic metastasis, as well as in lymphomas, where it is especially accurate in indicating extranodal disease, indicating appropriate therapy, therapeutic response and in indicating change in treatment.

BGO dedicated PET scanners, although expensive, have proved to be cost-effective. With a population catchment of 1 – 2 million, two scanners will have enough material to work at optimum level. Lower cost, lower performance alternatives, e.g. BGO partial-ring PET, NaI ring PET and NaI dual head gamma camera have a lower cost-benefit. High-performance PET scanners using new detector materials and configuration give a better performance and image quality. Dedicated systems for clinical PET are optimised for whole-body FDG studies. Though it costs less than current BGO PET, image quality is marginally better and is faster to use. PET – CT hybrid scanners give excellent images for practical application in planning therapy and monitoring response *(O'Doherty, M.J., Marsden, P.K.).*

Isotope Scanning

Advantages	Disadvantages
Access to a large number of body systems and organs with continuous development of new tracers.	Use of radioactive substances with obvious concerns to public.
Relative lack of reaction to intra-venous injection of radio-active tracer.	Relatively poor image resolution producing inadequate anatomical detail.
Significant information on functionality of body system, e.g., estimation of GFR, cardiac output, thyroid function.	Uptake of tracer in other organs producing some loss of detail and specificity.
Simple and easy on patients.	Disposal of radioactive waste could be problematic when using long half-life agents.

Figure 3.5 – *Advantages and disadvantages of Isotope Scanning.*

ERCP

This is a standard technique for diagnosing and sometimes treating a variety of pancreatic and biliary tract disorders. There are other invasive (e.g. PTC) and non-invasive (e.g. MRCP, CT, ultrasound, radionuclide liver-spleen scan), which may to some extent be considered competitive but often are complimentary.
Main indications for ERCP: (American Society for Gastroenterology – 1986)

1. Evaluation of persistent jaundice where biliary obstruction is suspected.
2. Evaluation of the non-jaundiced patient with suspected biliary tract disease, either intra- or extra- hepatic.
3. Suspected pancreatic cancer when prior imaging is normal or equivocal.
4. Recurrent pancreatitis of unknown aetiology.
5. Suspected pseudocyst of the pancreas with previous normal or equivocal imaging.

6. Pre-operative assessment of known pancreatic pseudocyst, chronic pancreatitis, or pancreatic trauma.

Main contraindications:
1. Patient refusal or poor cooperation.
2. Recent attack of pancreatitis unless undergoing endoscopic sphincterotomy or surgery.
3. Recent myocardial infarction.
4. Inadequate surgical backup.
5. History of contrast dye anaphylaxis.

Disadvantages:
1. Technically difficult.
2. Relatively hazardous.
3. Expensive.
4. Radiation exposure.

Magnetic Resonance Imaging

MRI uses the body's natural magnetic properties to produce images. The hydrogen nucleus (a single proton) is used because of its abundance in water and fat. When the body is placed in a strong magnetic field, the axis of the protons, which were previously randomly aligned, become aligned in the axis of the MRI scanner (magnetic vector). If radio wave frequency is added to the magnetic field, the magnetic vector is deflected. When the radio frequency source is switched off the magnetic vector returns to its resting state (relaxation), causing the emission of a radio wave signal. These signals are plotted in grey scale and cross sectional images built up as a series of pulse sequences. Different tissues have different relaxation times and can be identified.

Whole body MRI has been applied very effectively in oncology, principally in detecting skeletal secondaries and at the same time the soft tissue organs, so as to assess the total tumour burden. In the same way it can detect the primary tumour. It is also useful in the staging of tumours in pregnant patients. MRI has also non-oncological applications e.g. as an alternative to autopsies, for localizing percutaneous biopsies, for whole body fat measurements and in the diagnosis of polymyositis *(Nelson, E.)*.

Advantages	Disadvantages
High contrast spatial resolution in comparison with CT.	Very expensive.
The slice can be either sagittal or coronal (cf. CT Scan) without moving patient. i.e. any plane is possible.	Not so good for acute trauma (magnetic effect on support apparatus).
No ionising radiation.	Not so useful for lungs, cortical bone and hollow abdominal organs.
No bone artefacts.	Less effective for regions prone to motion.
Allows better differentiation of tissue types including cancer staging e.g. rectal cancer, indicating need for pre-op DXT.	Slower than Spiral CT or Multislice Scanner.
Allows non-invasive vascular imaging without iodine-based contrast agents.	Contraindicated in the presence of pacemakers and certain metallic implants.
Allows functional imaging with spectroscopy and diffusion studies.	
Superior to CT for soft tissue, bone marrow, pelvic organs and cerebral imaging except for trauma.	

Figure 3.6 – *Advantages and disadvantages of Magnetic Resonance Imaging.*

Magnetic Resonance Cholangiopancreatography (MRCP)

This is an application of MRI to biliary and pancreatic ducts. The pancreatic and biliary anatomy is shown with a sharpness similar to direct contrast cholangiopancreatography. It is a non-invasive alternative to diagnostic ERCP.

Advantages	Disadvantages
Non-invasive (Avoids complications of diagnostic ERPC and PTC).	Not widely available at high quality.
No sedation usually required.	Is superfluous if therapeutic ERCP is necessary.
No ionising radiation.	Duct images may be obscured by other fluid structures eg renal cysts, pseudocysts or ascites.
No iodinated intravenous contrast medium used.	Contraindicated in the presence of ferromagnetic implants.
Rapid scan time.	Other implants may cause artefacts.
Delineates anatomy proximal to obstructions.	Claustrophobic.
Delineates anatomy post biliary-enteric anastomosis.	Lack of standardized scanning protocols.
T1 images define extraductal structures e.g. lymph nodes, vascular structures, metastasis, which is useful for staging.	

Figure 3.7– *Advantages and disadvantages of MRCP compared with ERCP.*

Ultrasound Scanning

Advantages	Disadvantages
Simple and safe without the use of radiation.	Totally dependent on operator as mainly a real time procedure (most procedures are 'operator dependent').
Flexible and covers many regions of the body.	Optimal images dependent on good patient preparation e.g. full bladder in pelvic scan.
High tissue specificity with high quality machines.	Limitation with fat overweight patients since sound is easily attenuated by adipose tissues.
Real time examination with ability to view anatomy/pathology in different planes just by rotation of the probe.	Attenuation of sound by bowel gas.
Ability to assess vascular pathology using Doppler and colour Doppler techniques.	Sophisticated equipment is relatively expensive, especially individual probes.
Aid for image guided interventional techniques like percutaneous nephrostomy and biopsy.	
Use in intra-operative procedures to help with greater access to disease.	

Figure 3.8 – *Advantages and disadvantages of Ultrasound Scanning (Crockford, M.).*

Bone Mineral Density Scan

The energy of X-ray beams, usually using two different energies, that passes through bones and what is not absorbed can be detected and measured on the other side of the body. The greater the mineral content of the bones, which makes the bones more dense, allows less X-ray energy to pass through. Knowing the penetrating energy per pixel, the number of pixels in the area and the amount of bone in each pixel, allows the bone density to be calculated. Bone density is recorded as T-scores (related to average peak bone mass), or Z-scores (related to bone mass depending on age). T-sores less than 2.5 indicates osteoporosis. Z-scores are useful for long-term follow-up.

Advantages	Disadvantages
Basic measurements are quickly done.	Metal objects (including piercing) are a source of error.
Two energy beams allow estimates for soft tissues separate from those of bones.	Radiation dose is 1.5 times that of a Chest X-ray.
Measurements may be taken in A-P or lateral views.	

Figure 3.9 *(Berger, A.)*

Interventional Radiology

Advantages	Disadvantages
Additional range of interventions possible in the treatment of difficult clinical problems.	Dangerous if not carried out by experienced radiologists trained specifically in these techniques.
Use of local rather than general anaesthetic in procedures reduces risks.	Needs close interaction of clinical colleagues and nursing staff who will understand and follow up problems that could arise.
Use of imaging facilities to access more directly and accurately the clinical area required.	Needs special budget to acquire range of consumables that are often very expensive. E.g. Vena Cava filters cost around Lm500.
Relative lack of complications since smaller needles, blades and other instruments used.	Needs to be carried out in an imaging environment.
Often considered as a first step in treatment of some clinical situation. E.g. Percutaneous nephrostomy to improve renal function.	Carried out in close conjunction with clinician, who may decide to deal operatively with the situation if interventional technique fails.
Sometimes used to aid subsequent surgery and help improve results. E.g. iliac artery angioplasty followed by fem-pop graft, pre-op embolisation of renal tumours to reduce vascular field.	
Day case interventions reducing hospital stay and thus costs to the health service.	

Figure 3.10 – *Advantages and disadvantages of Interventional Radiology (Crockford, M.).*

The complexity and expense of the technology, the numerous options available in determining a plan of diagnostic study and the variation in expense, safety and efficacy of the various modalities available, should entice the clinician to adopt a less dictatorial attitude in requesting such special investigations. Help is needed to choose the most practical, prompt and cost-effective imaging investigation to request, in order to achieve the goal in management of the case. The radiologist must become more involved in the care of the patient, at least in so far as the ends of the patient's management are concerned. With increased complexity of the technology, even the help of a committed radiologist might not be sufficient, and he might have to act as a middleman between the pure scientist and technician on one hand and the clinician and patient on the other, serving as a catalyst between these two groups *(James, E.A. et al.)*

The clinician should not blush at these suggestions exhorting a sharing of decision making in management of his patients, when so much is at stake.

Histopathological Investigations

The histopathologist provides tissue diagnosis, he often gives helpful information leading to appropriate planning of the patient's future management and better assessment of his prognosis e.g. in staging and grading malignant neoplasms. Staging also allows comparisons and assessment of therapies, comparing apples with apples. With advances in molecular biology, new imaging techniques and more selective surgical procedures e.g. sentinel node biopsies, more realistic and accurate staging allows tailored therapeutic decisions for particular tumour and host characteristics. Through a post-mortem examination, he may help the clinician to understand the disease process and to correlate symptoms and signs with the pathological changes.

The surgeon must communicate well with the pathologist and understand his requirements. The reverse also holds. A pathologist must communicate well with his colleagues as well as the clinicians, advise about the biopsy material he receives, the extent of the disease, grade of malignancy, adequacy of the excision, prognosis and possibly the need for further therapy. The pathological report essentially consists of five parts:

The 1st part contains the main clinical data including any past histology report.

The 2nd part describes the specimen grossly.

The 3rd part contains a short description of the microscopic appearance.

The 4th contains the pathological diagnosis.

The 5th contains the pathologist's comments, variably regarding differential diagnosis, prognosis and occasionally therapeutic implications e.g. ER status, excision margins.

Consultation with other pathologists is in everybody's interest especially the patient's. This is made easier by modern technology e.g. telemedicine. Pathologists have the same potential for error as other medical practitioners.

Biopsy techniques are often essential in diagnosis especially in oncology. Several methods are used, including incisional biopsy, excisional biopsy, endoscopic biopsy, core needle biopsy and fine needle aspiration. Incisional biopsies imply that only a portion of the lesion is sampled and it can only be of diagnostic value. When excisional biopsies are done the whole lesion is excised usually with a rim of normal tissue. The other biopsy techniques are self-explanatory. Whichever method is used, an adequate volume of tissue allows the use of various specialised techniques e.g. various fixatives, histochemical studies, bioassay or tissue culture. These may prove to be essential in difficult cases. If the tissue submitted to the pathologist is inadequate for confident interpretation, it is the pathologist's duty to say so rather than risk a dreadful mistake. In the rare case of an insoluble problem, the pathologist suggests a differential diagnosis, which the clinician can usefully confront with the clinical picture.

One can enumerate several points, which are important for the surgeon who is considering taking biopsy material:

(i)   The larger the lesion, the more numerous the (non-excisional) biopsies should be, because the pathology may be focal or variable.

(ii) In ulcerated lesions, the biopsies should be taken from the periphery, including both abnormal and normal tissues.

(iii) A biopsy taken from too peripheral a site may only show reactive inflammation.

(iv) The biopsy should be deep enough so that the relationship between the pathology and stroma can be seen.

(v) All fragments removed must be sent to the pathology lab and examined.

(vi) Crushing and squeezing of specimens causes artefacts and should be avoided.

(vii) The biopsy material should be placed immediately in an adequate volume of fixative (about ten times the volume of the tissue one wants to fix).

(viii) Specimen labelling should be meticulous.

(ix) Depending on the type of pathological examination requested, one must use the correct fixative e.g. specimens for frozen section should not be sent in formol-salne.

(x) The specimens should be sent in optimum time.

(xi) Depending on the known or presumed nature of the pathology, one may consider and take all necessary steps to request special studies e.g. electron microscopy, genomic studies *(Rosai, J.)*.

Frozen Section

One may reasonably request this technique:

(a) To establish the presence and nature of a lesion when urgent knowledge of the pathology will influence the course of the operation.

(b) To determine the adequacy of the surgical margins.

(c) To establish whether the sampling has diagnosable material or more sampling is necessary.

The limitations of frozen section vary according to the organ involved. Good communication between clinician and pathologist, regarding the clinical background and indications for using the technique is even more crucial for the successful outcome of this special investigation. The possible answer forthcoming from the pathologist may be that the pathology is benign, that it is malignant, or the pathologist may declare that he or she is not sure and that the decision has to be deferred till examination of the routine H and E sections are examined. An abundance of statistical evaluations regarding this technique have been published over the years. An average of 17 studies is as follows:

Accuracy.............96%

False positives.......0.24%

False negatives......1.87%

Deferred..............1.76%

(Oneson, R.H., Minke, J.A., Silverber, S.G.)

Diagnostic Cytology

When performed by an experienced cytologist, a positive cytological diagnosis is as reliable as a tissue biopsy. False positives in these circumstances hardly ever occur. False negatives also depend on the source of the material.

In most organs a cytological diagnosis should be confirmed by a tissue biopsy, even though experienced operators give reliable results. Thus, in most clinical scenarios, one would confirm a positive FNA result on a breast lump, with a core biopsy, in addition to consideration of other diagnostic modalities such as clinical findings and mammography and/or breast ultrasound, before embarking on major surgery. An exception to this statement is a positive bronchial carcinoma cytology in a patient with radiological evidence of bronchial carcinoma. This latter situation is considered sufficient evidence to justify a decision on therapy.

There are several practical considerations regarding the use of this technique *(Hajdu, S.I., Melamed, M.R.):*

1. Aspiration cytology should not be use in preference to larger biopsies when the latter can be easily and safely obtained.
2. In FNA samples the architecture is lost and it is not possible to clinch a diagnosis that is based on histology.
3. Cytological diagnosis must correlate with the clinical data. The latter information is essential for the cytologist.
4. The cytological diagnosis of malignancy is simpler than its classification.
5. Only positive findings give real information.
6. Negative reports should lead to more clinical probing and/or more investigative procedures.
7. Unwarranted use of FNA serves only to discredit a useful but not universally applicable, technique.

Dynamic Investigations

Electrophysiology offers good examples of dynamic testing. Here, what matters is the propagation of action potentials in nerves and muscles, the efficacy of the neuromuscular interface and the effectiveness of sensory transaction. The measurement of electrical potential as a function of time provides this information.

Consultation

The investigative process may come to a point where the opinion of a colleague in the same or other speciality is clearly indicated. If the case is an urgent one a personal approach is by far preferable to an impersonal consultation form sent through hospital mail. In less urgent situations, an informative, condensed letter delivered by hand to the receiver (having made sure the person is available and perhaps supplementing it with a telephone message) may be sufficient.

Post-mortem Examinations

Though a post-mortem exam should ideally be performed on each hospital death, this is hardly attainable for logistic reasons. When the cause of death is unknown, the demise unexpected, or there are legal or medico-legal indications, the relatives should be approached tactfully and sympathetically and requested to consent to an autopsy. If the practical reasons are explained the relatives will usually comply *(Kyle, J.)*. In case of refusal, an on-call magistrate (in Malta) should be informed after notifying the consultant in charge of the case, if he is not already directly involved, and a magisterial inquiry and post-mortem will be held. By law, 'violent deaths' and death due to unknown cause have to take the latter course.

Investigations for Screening

Historically, screening programs were intended for the detection, prevention and control of communicable diseases. Present screening programmes are mainly directed at neoplasia, more specifically breast, cervical and gastric cancer. This shift in emphasis towards screening and, hopefully, early detection, of malignant neoplasia is understandable considering that in western Europe today a third of the population develop a malignancy at least once in their lifetime *(Lindblom, A., Linjegren, A.)* and cancer is responsible for a quarter of all deaths.

Current Screening Programmes

Disease	Screening Modality	Comments
Breast cancer	Self-examination, clinical examination, mammography.	The age group, which seems to benefit is 50-69 years. Younger women do not seem to benefit. Older age groups have been insufficiently researched.
Colorectal cancer	Faecal occult blood, sigmoidoscopy.	Reduces death rate. Opportunistic screening of high-risk groups is even more effective.
Gastric cancer	Endoscopic examination.	Early detection and increased cure rates in Japan.
Prostatic cancer	DRE and PSA.	Optimal therapy for early prostatic cancer is not defined. The impact of screening for cancer of the prostate has not been ascertained by RCT's. More intensive screening by serum PSA and prostatic biopsy, as well as more frequent use of DXT and radical prostatectomy in proved cases, do not lower the mortality over an 11 year period. (Lou-Yao G et al.)
Uterine cervix	Exfoliative cytology.	Detects sqamous cell carcinoma but not adenocarcinoma. The latter constitutes 15% of cervical cancers.
Ovarian cancer	Serum CA-125 or trans-vaginal ultrasound.	Not enough evidence to support screening.
Lung cancer	Chest X-Ray, sputum cytology.	No reduction in mortality even if opportunistic screening in high-risk groups is done.

Figure 3.11

Screening programs separate the population into a high-risk group, which requires further investigation to confirm or exclude the presence of the disease, and a group which is unlikely to have the disease. Detection of disease requires a test with a high sensitivity while its exclusion requires investigations with a high specificity (vide Chapter 3 earlier on).

The advisability of adoption of screening programmes is often dominated by advocacy from pressure groups rather than from scientific debate. However, justification of a screening programme should involve certain requirements. These criteria were originally put forward by the WHO *(Wilson and Yungner)* focusing on chronic diseases. These criteria may, however, interact and should not be considered individually. Essentially these include:

(i) The disease must have a high incidence.

(ii) It must have serious consequences.

(iii) The natural history of the disease should be well understood, making it possible to be detected in an early pre-clinical phase before it spreads.

(iv) Treatment of the disease after early detection should produce significant benefit.

(v) Availability of a suitable investigative method, which is easily reproducible, acceptable to the patient and of acceptable cost-benefit *(Sweetland, H.M., Monypenny, I.J.)*.

It has been suggested that when evaluating screening for genetic susceptibility, the above criteria may have to be marginally modified. These include: a good knowledge of the characteristics of the population proposed to be studied, the need for valid and acceptable methods for identifying those individuals in the target population who are going to benefit from such testing, the knowledge of the risks involved, knowledge of the course from susceptibility to the pre-clinical phase, and including social and psychological costs to the financial ones *(Goel V. for Crossroads 99 Group)*.

Screening programmes have their disadvantages, which include the patient's anxiety, false positive and false negative results, over-diagnosis and over-treatment, physical adverse effects and cost. Also, because of the complexity of tumour growth and the frequent rapid dissemination, screening may not live up to its theoretical promise. Early detection of tumour need not necessarily mean detection of early tumour. In other words, a clinically 'early' tumour need not be biologically early, i.e. in its natural history or behaviour. For example, in a study involving almost 40,000 women aged from 50 to 59 years (Canadian Breast Screening Study), mammography was found to detect breast cancer earlier than physical examination but this did not translate into a survival advantage. The probable explanation is that mammography is more effective for detecting lesions of low malignant potential. In addition earlier detection by mammography wanes off the longer the period of follow-up. In other words, careful physical breast examination is as effective as mammographic screening in reducing the mortality from breast cancer. This has been confirmed by another large study involving more than 50,000 volunteers which were followed up for 11 to 16 years *(Miller, A.B. et al.)*: In the 40 to 49 year age group, annual mammography combined with self examination and 4 to 5 annual clinical examination, did not improve the death rate from breast cancer when compared with the usual community care, a single clinical examination and instruction on self examination. There have been two more recent publications comparing mortalities before and after mammographic screening was introduced, which both point towards a reduction in mortality. The first *(Taber, L. et al.)* compares death from breast cancer in two Swedish counties 20 years before mammography screening every 18 months, with that after the programme started. This study involved 210,000 women and resulted in an adjusted death risk drop of 23%. In the 40 – 49 year age group, there was a drop of 48%. One notes that there was also a drop in death risk of 19% even in women that were not screened. The second study involved the age group 55 - 74 years *(Otto, S.J. et al.)*: The mortality in 2001 was 20% lower than in1986 - 1988 i.e. before mammography screening was instituted. This translates into an average reduction in mortality of 1.7% compared wit a previous trend for a 0.3% increase per year. Though one must note these results, the potential for biases in these studies is obvious. Considering the lack of convincing evidence in favour of breast cancer screening and the potential harm that may result from it e.g. unnecessary interventions and anxiety, there seems to be little scientific justification for the vociferous support it receives from pressure groups.

Another danger in screening for cancer is over-diagnosis bias. This results in a difference between survival and mortality data, in that survival data are effected whilst mortality data are not. This has been shown in screening trials for lung cancer *(Marcus, P. et al : Mayo Lung Project)*. Other studies investigating screening for lung cancer *(Wolpaw, D.R.)* and prostate cancer *(Kranse, R. et al.) (Parkes, C. et al.)* show that diagnosis of earlier lesions by screening, did not result in better outcomes for the screened group when compared with the control group. This is probably because low grade (rather than early) tumours which would never have presented clinically, are detected by screening. The same consideration applies to mammography. The GMC guidelines state that women undergoing breast screening should be informed of the drawbacks of mammography as well as the potential benefits. The efficacy of mammography and regular PSA estimations for screening breast and prostate cancer respectively has been questioned basing on systematic reviews. *(Charatan, F.)*. This provoked a reaction, which was as irate as it was poorly justified. One wonders whether financial considerations were a possible factor in provoking this response.

When considering prostate cancer, screening could be relevant in 4 groups:
1. The cases that present and are diagnosed clinically. At present, outcome is not affected by treatment and therefore screening cannot help.
2. Rapidly progressive cancer. Screening does not improve outcome.
3. Screening-identified cancer which would never have become symptomatic or relevant in the patient's lifetime. There is a possibility of unnecessary treatment.
4. Asymptomatic individuals, diagnosed by screening, whose disease can be helped by treatment and would have otherwise have progressed beyond the scope of treatment. It is desirable to identify this group, but with our present methods this is difficult.

If one were to consider one million men over 50 years, one would statistically expect:

110,000 to have a raised PSA.

90,000 will undergo prostatic biopsy.

20,000 will be diagnosed as having prostatic cancer.

10,000 will undergo surgery.

Over 4,000 will have impotence.

300 will develop severe urinary incontinence.

10 will die in the peri-operative period.

Only 16% of patients diagnosed as having prostatic cancer by screening benefit from radical surgery. *(McGregor, et al.)* On the other hand, men are more likely to die with, rather than from carcinoma of the prostate. One concludes that at present, national programmes for prostatic cancer screening are not justified *(Frankel, S. et al.)*.

When considering screening for colorectal cancer, the mortality risks of the disease in those screened by sigmoidoscopy are 25% of those who are not screened. (Newcomb P et al.). This reduction seems to be sustained for 15 years, probably because a polyp takes as long as 15 years to undergo malignant change. More research with RTC's is required to give more reliable indications as to the time intervals of sigmoidoscopies and colonoscopies.

It has been calculated that in the NHS cervical screening programme, 1,000 women need to be screened for 35 years to prevent a single cervical cancer death *(Raffle, A.E. et al.)*. One must take also into account the possible harmful effects resulting from cervical cancer screening e.g. over-detection, iatrogenic harm from invasive investigation and treatment, doubts about the progression from dysplasia to malignancy and the necessity to assure an acceptable level of accuracy of the programme.

Yet another example is provided by the more recent issue of whole body CT screening for cancer. In fact there is no proven benefit for this screening procedure. Furthermore, serious risks could outweigh any possible benefits, resulting in unnecessary surgery for benign nodules. In this context there are some interesting statistics: The false positive rate of this form of screening is high, amounting to 70% of all participants *(Swensen, S.J.)*. 50% of all lung nodules removed at surgery are benign *(Bernard, A.)*. Mortality from this type of surgical procedure is 3.8% *(Romano, P.S. et al.)*. The financial cost of this 'screening' procedure is high, amounting to 2.3 million USD per quality-adjusted life year gained *(Mahadevia, P.J. et al.)*.

One assumes that a similar bias can occur during screening for other types of cancer, though this has not been scientifically demonstrated. It is also possible that more sophisticated and precise investigative procedures used in screening, e.g. spiral CT, may allow distinction of the relevant pathologies and therefore improve the results of screening. This is, however, far from sure. One need not stress that tumour size is no guide to tumour age or aggressiveness.

When effective, cancer screening should result in a shifting of the distribution curve towards a prevalence of less advanced cases, prolonged survival and lower mortality in the screened population. The latter is the best evidence of the success of the screening method and is best estimated using randomised controlled trials comparing mortality from the disease in the general non-screened population with that of the screened group. One should take care to eliminate lead-time bias (bringing forward the date at which the diagnosis is made), length bias (detection of disproportion of slow-growing tumours) and selection bias (attraction of more health conscious and better socio-economic status groups). The designing and running of these trials is not easy, as is evidenced by the confusion and contradictions of results of breast screening trials *(Gotzsche, P.C. and Olsen, O.)*. The method of randomisation and possible changes in numbers, design and analysis should be clearly specified *(de Koning, H.J.)*.

One may decide to test a patient or a group of patients for a particular disease when they are considered to be particularly at risk, because of their symptoms, past medical history, family history or social history. An example is provided by the influence of family history on the incidence of carcinoma of the breast: If the sister or mother had the disease, the chances of the patient developing carcinoma of the breast increases to 2 to 3 times normal. If both mother and sister had breast cancer, the chances of the patient developing the same malignancy increase six-fold. This statistic is even more alarming if the relatives had developed the cancer at an early age. Thus one may decide to target such high-risk groups in what is termed opportunistic screening, in contradistinction to population screening. This may be associated with improved cost benefit and efficacy.

Conclusion

'Data, give me data!' expostulated Sherlock Holmes.

Intelligent and efficient collection of data i.e. the best available clinical evidence, is only a basis for analysis and application of such vital data to patient management. Anything falling outside these guidelines is futile, wasteful and sometimes even dangerous and cruel.

Chapter 4

Surgical Treatment

The essence of our profession is to be of service to others. While disease may or may not be curable, a doctor's duty is to help others through commitment, compassion, care, the desire to learn and improve and pass our knowledge to others.

Quotations:
Hippocrates – Greek physician; Father of Medicine (ca. 460 – 337 BC):
'We ought not to reject the ancient Art, as if it were not and had not been properly founded, because it did not attain accuracy in all things, but rather, since it is capable of reaching to the greatest exactitude by reasoning, to receive it and admire its discoveries, made from a state of great ignorance, and as having been well and properly made and not from chance'.

'The patient.......may recover his health simply through his contentment with the goodness of his physician'.

The Sage of Cos

'I would define (the aims of) Medicine as the complete removal of the distress of the sick, the alleviation of the more violent diseases, and the refusal to undertake to cure cases in which the disease has already won the mastery'.

Document of the Burial Society Herwah Kaddishah - Josefov Ceremonial Hall (Prague):
Medicine in the Ghetto (1564)
'Sickness represents both Divine visitation and the call to help one's fellow beings. This is why medical intervention to heal the sick is not seen as a negation of the will of God, but as a religious duty'.

Voltaire (1694 – 1778) – French writer and philosopher:
'The art of medicine consists of amusing the patient while nature cures the disease'.

Edward Harrison – British physician (1766 – 1830):
'The practising physician must never forget that his primary and traditional objectives are utilitarian, - the prevention and cure of disease and the relief of suffering, whether in body or in mind'.

Sir Howard Florey – British pathologist and Nobel laureate (1898 – 1968):
'The main reason why a patient sees a doctor is to be relieved of his symptoms. His medical attendant endeavours to do this by therapeutic procedures directed to relieving the symptoms or, more rationally to dealing with the underlying cause'.

Sir William Osler – Canadian-American physician (1849 – 1919):

'From Hippocrates to Hunter the treatment of disease was one long traffic in hypothesis'.

Sir Berkeley Moynihan – British surgeon (1865 –1936):

'The surgeon may in some degree share his responsibility with others, but the chief responsibility must always lie with him, and being his, must be exercised not only during the operation but also before, perhaps long before, and also after, perhaps long after, the operation is performed'.

Sir Robert Hutchinson – British paediatrician (1871 – 1960):

'From inability to leave well alone,
From too much zeal for what is new and contempt for what is old,
From putting knowledge before wisdom,
Science before art,
Cleverness before common sense,
From treating patients as cases, and
From making the cure of the disease more grievous
than its endurance,
Good Lord, deliver us'.

Dr.V.L. Ackerman – Pathologist, St. Louis, Missouri, U.S.A. –1905-1993.

'A good surgeon has not only technical dexterity,(a fairly common commodity), but also, more importantly, good judgement and a personal concern for his patients' welfare. The surgeon with a prepared mind and a clear concept of the pathology of disease, invariably is one with good judgement'.

The Hippocratic Oath

'I swear by Apollo, the physician, and Aesculapius, and Health, and All-Heal, and all the gods and goddesses, that according to my ability and judgement, I shall keep this oath and stipulation:

1. To reckon him who taught me this art as equally dear to me as my parents.

2. To share my substance with him and relieve his necessities if required.

3. To regard his offspring as on the same footing as my own brothers.

4. To teach them this art if they should wish to learn it, without fee or stipulation.

5. With every method I shall impart a knowledge of the art to my sons, and those of my teachers, and to disciples bound by stipulation and oath, according to the law of medicine, but to none others.

6. I shall follow that method of treatment which, according to my ability and judgement, I consider for the benefit of my patients, and abstain from what is deleterious and mischievous.

7. I shall give no deadly medicine to anyone if asked, nor suggest any such counsel.

8. I shall not give a woman an instrument to produce abortion.

9. With purity and holiness I shall pass my life and practice my art.

10. I shall not cut a person who is suffering from stone, but will leave this to be done by practitioners of this work.

11. I shall enter houses for the benefit of the sick and abstain from every voluntary act of mischief and corruption and from seduction of females or males, slaves or free.

12. I shall keep secret whatever I may see or hear of the lives of men in connection with my profession

or otherwise.

13. While I continue to keep this oath may it be granted to me to enjoy life and the practice of this art, respected by all men at all time; but should I violate this oath may the reverse be my lot'.

Surgical Decision Making

One would desire to be always provided with undeniable data from which one can conclude logical (and hopefully useful) surgical decisions. This is wishful thinking since:

a) Hardly ever is a single symptom, sign or test pathognomonic,

b) Matters are rarely absolute in clinical decisions. Surgical decisions are almost always estimates of probabilities and balancing trade-offs. They are consequently subject to error.

Surgical decision making is not only potentially difficult of its own nature, but has become even more so due to the following circumstances:

a) The scope of Surgery has increased enormously, with an increased potential for investigation and treatment.

b) Pressure from society.

    (i)   Increased need for surgical investigation and treatment partly due to the increase in life expectancy.
    (ii)   Increased public awareness (the media).
    (iii)   Cost constraints on the delivery of health care.
    (iv)   The rights of the individual patient.
    (v)   Political considerations.
    (vi)   Medico-legal considerations.
    (vii) Ethical considerations.

c) Limitations of Surgical Training

    (i)   Limited time - Trainees aspire to become Consultants as soon as possible and indeed cannot be limited to training posts for too long. Training schemes have been worked out by the Colleges and other bodies. Working hours have become more reasonable in recent years. Though entirely reasonable, this has limited time for training even further. Better planning and increased efficacy of training can only in part make up for this.
    (ii)   Limited access to training posts due to logistic and financial constraints.
    (iii)   Enormous volume of material, ever increasing, which needs to be absorbed: The knowledge base for a clinician is over 15 million facts and increasing

daily. The number of such facts one can learn and retain is about 9 facts per hour, i.e. it should take a trainee almost one million, seven hundred thousand hours or one hundred and ninety four years of continuous, completely efficient study to absorb this material. This is obviously impossible and one has to accept one's limitations and increase efficiency to its maximum.

Management of the Surgical Patient - General Considerations

The approach to surgical management follows certain steps with the clinician facing the following questions:

A) What is the problem?

B) What are the available options?
   (i)   Return patient to the family doctor.
   (ii)   Do nothing and review later.
   (iii) Investigate and review later.
   (iv)   As in (iii) but institute conservative therapy.
   (v)   As in (iv) but prepare patient physically and mentally
          for possible operation.
   (vi)   Immediate operation.

C) Selecting the best option.

D) Assessing patient's preferences, values, consent and rights.

E) Actions to be taken
   (i)   Urgently
   (ii)   On a routine basis.

F) Ascertaining compliance when treatment plan is done by patient independently.

One has to realise that medical knowledge is often probabilistic. Often one cannot be absolutely sure what is the best treatment, for the most likely diagnosis, in a particular patient, though one knows roughly the probability of the diagnosis and likelihood of cure with the particular treatment. This leads to divergent opinions on treatment on occasions. A clinician can often offer informed advice on treatment and not certainty and this reflects also his own attitudes and experience. In an attempt to have a more scientific basis for such advice and surgical decisions, risk scores have been proposed e.g. for upper GIT haemorrhage, where clinical, endoscopic and laboratory variables are taken into account.

Another example illustrating this problem is the controversy surrounding the pathogenesis, risk of malignancy and management of Barrett's oesophagus: The risk of malignancy in cases having Barrett's oesophagus is said to be 0.5% per year, which is about 30 times that in the general population. This would seem to be a very clear indication for aggressive therapy for this condition if this therapy is safe, convenient and the expense is reasonable. There are, however, some other relevant considerations: Barrett's oesophagus may be subdivided into a 'long-segment' variety, which is more than 3 centimetres long and occurs in 3-5% of GORD, and the 'short-segment' variety which is more than 3 centimetres and is found in 10-15% of cases of GORD at OGD. It is not clear whether these have the same pathogenesis or carry the same risks of malignancy. Furthermore, survival of Barrett's oesophagus cases is the same as that for the general population. The latter statistic may result from the high percentage of old people, who have high co-morbidity, involved in these studies. An even more forceful argument is that even if there were a highly effective cancer-preventive treatment for Barrett's oesophagus, it would take 400 such patients to be treated to prevent one single case of oesophageal cancer in one year *(Spelcher, S.J.)*. Despite all these arguments, regular endoscopic surveillance is the only management strategy that is widely recommended. These recommendations are based on observational studies which are subject to several biases such as lead time, length time and selection bias, and computer models which depend on their baseline assumptions. The other side of the coin is that failing to perform an endoscopy may result in missing an adenocarcinoma of the oesophagus at a potentially curable stage.

Patient Involvement in Clinical Decision Making

It has become fashionable to propose systems where patients play an important role decision making about management. Doctors are, quite rightly, expected to share their knowledge, or lack of it, with their patients, whilst the latter are given access to background information on disease and health issues. There are two factors which influence this issue:

The first is patient information. Aids have been evolved to help patients' involvement in decision making. These may take the form of simple charts, animated graphics, audio-narration and interactive computer technology. Providing these aids on internet reduces costs, improve access and the ease of updating. These improve patients' knowledge, reduce decisional conflict and stimulate the patient to take a more active part in the management of his own condition. There is no evidence that this eventually improves patient satisfaction. Even with the best of intentions, patient information leading to decision making is frequently insufficient. In the United States, where medico-legal and financial factors encourage maximal patient information, it has been calculated that in 17% of basic decisions, none of the intermediate decisions, and only 0.5% of complex decisions were patients completely informed *(Larkin M.)*. Patient information is a factor in management decisions. If patients are to participate actively in decisions about their health, they must be accurately and effectively informed in a simple form which the patient can surely assimilate (Plate 5.). The information must be based on the best available evidence and presented in a form that is acceptable and useful. Patient centred care means taking into account the patient's desire for information and sharing in decision making, which should then influence the resultant course of action *(Stewart, M.)*. It is doubtful whether the present surge of patient information via internet health related websites is a help, since the material is difficult to digest and sometimes inaccurate.

Plate 5

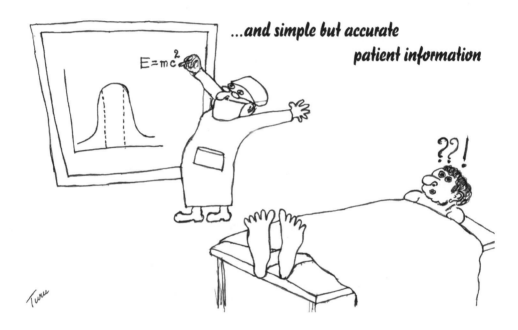

...and simple but accurate patient information

The second factor is patient safety. This may limit patient's choice if the alternatives are not equally safe, effective or reliable. One has to concede that particular concepts of safety may vary with time and circumstance. Thus, for example, the concept of pre-operative patient starvation have varied from the traditional withholding of food and drink from midnight before operation to more recent evidence that light meals may be allowed up to 4-6 hours and clear fluids up to 2 hours before induction of anaesthesia.

Placing the onus of a clinical decision entirely on the patient, even with the help of the above-mentioned aids, is a form of abdication of clinical responsibility, which is not likely to be in the patients' best interest. No amount of pre-digested information can improve on the clinical acumen, accumulated over years of sweat and blood, of a reliable clinician. This does not mean that patients should never be involved in clinical decision making. Good communication is a most important factor in the clinical rapport and there are indications that when patients are involved, the outcomes, especially subjective ones, improve. However, when weighting the patient's opinion on clinical management and decision making, one should consider a factor, which expresses the patient's knowledge of the problem, the background data necessary in the patient's possession and also the patient's personal ability regarding decision making. Patients may favour an investigative or a therapeutic option because of insufficient or incorrect data, or else poor processing of correct data. Yielding to, or compromising with, such pressures from patients could lead to untenable situations, such as the impressively high caesarean section rate in some South American countries *(De Mello, E., Souza, C.)*. This particular example may in part be due to the fact that caesarean section may be more convenient and financially rewarding for the doctors, who then present encouraging data to the patient in favour of caesarean section. This data then circulates amongst the general public. Communication includes patient information about risks of the proposed or alternative forms of management so as to avoid unrealistic expectations. Treatment, however, should not be denied, or a 'refusal' suggested simply because of risk.

The way doctors communicate information has been traditionally classed into three approaches: (i) A paternalistic approach where one uses short descriptions of physical symptoms, leading to diagnostic categories without giving much importance to patients' values and concerns. (ii) An informed approach where relevant information from research and personal experience is discussed with the patient, who can then make an informed decision. (iii) A shared approach involving an interactive relationship with the patients. In fact these theoretical subdivisions hardly ever occur in their ideal form. The preponderance of one or other of these approaches varies depending on different factors e.g. the patient's intelligence, age, trust, psychological consistency etc. In the most favourable circumstances, shared decision making may improve the doctor patient relationship in some cases, but may result in great insecurity and anxiety in others. It is conceivable to apply decision analysis so as to include patients' preferences and values in the process of clinical decision making, when there is good and clear clinical evidence, which is thoroughly understood by the right type of patient. Doctors need to possess the skills and thorough knowledge of their patients, so as to decide who of these, and at which level, would prefer to be involved in decisions on medical management. One also needs the time, patience and intellect to realise when it is in the patient's interest. Deciding which patients to involve in such processes is the burden of the clinician and is not less onerous than taking the responsibility for the clinical decision itself.

The issue of patient involvement in clinical decision making becomes more complex when one considers the problems involved in advanced directives, impaired capacity and surrogate decision making. The medical situation and the consequent care-needs, almost invariably, present a state of flux rather than a static situation. Surrogate decisions may well reflect the views of the surrogate rather than those of the patient they are deciding for. In this way a complex situation is rendered superficially simpler but less transparent, just or even ethical.

Telemedicine

Telemedicine, sometimes called online health or e-health, refers to any medical activity where there is an element of distance. This has taken the form of home tele nursing, teleradiology, electronic referrals to specialists and hospitals, teleconsultations between general practitioners and specialists, minor injuries telemedicine for nurses, health information centres and online health. However, there is little evidence for its clinical and cost effectiveness. Its main indication is where benefit to patients e.g. quicker access to appropriate expertise, avoidance of commuting, outweigh its disadvantages, such as, costs. The health sector must learn how to make the best use of this and other technologies. It may require changes in attitude and in delivery practices *(Wooton R)*.

In developing countries, telemedicine has the potential of having an impact on several aspects of health care. When implementing such a technology, one has to consider the historical, cultural and technological peculiarities, including the infrastructure, of the region concerned, as well as the inherent disadvantages that such systems carry.

Clinical Decision Making

Correct data and information, on its own does not suffice for effective decision making. It is also important that the data is delivered in a digestible and useful form and that the 'user' is competent to elaborate the data and derive logical conclusions. The background needed for this competence is very vast (vide. 'Enormous volume of material' discussed previously) and this is the Achilles' tendon of the argument in favour of participation of the patient in clinical decision making on an equal footing with the clinician.

In surgery one of the most common and crucial dilemmas is the decision to operate. There are four basic questions one asks in these circumstances.
1. Is the pathology helped by operative treatment?
2. Is the pathology in the particular patient an indication for surgery?
3. Do the potential benefits outweigh the risks, in the particular patient? (Risk-benefit analysis).
4. Does the patient consent to the operative treatment advised?

It is well to recall that the aims of surgery are to:
(i)   Maintain life

(ii) Prolong life

(iii) Relieve or abolish pain

(iv) Improve or restore function

(v) Improve the quality of life

(vi) Establish diagnosis or stage disease.

One is justified in pursuing these aims when doing this is considered to be beneficial to the particular patient, having of course, ascertained the patient's informed consent.

Scoring Systems

Scoring systems have been developed to allocate priorities for operations e.g. Priority criteria for Cardiac Surgery (Hadorn DC, Holmes AC). These studies do not distinguish between 'priority' and 'urgency', and also fail to take the efficacy of the procedure into consideration. 'Urgency' is the speed required to obtain the desired clinical outcome, while 'priority' deals with the relative position on a surgical waiting list. Thus scoring systems may be useful in indicating that a particular patient deserves the operation, but not whether the operation is likely to help. In addition to their use in clinical management, scoring systems can also be for audit of comparable groups e.g. to compare different providers, and for research comparing outcomes e.g. to aid stratification in randomised controlled studies as well as for adjusting for differences in case mix. Scoring systems may be specific e.g. the Glasgow coma scale or the Revised Trauma Score, or generic e.g. the Apache I, II or III scale (Acute Physiology And Chronic Health Evaluation) *(Gunning, K.E.J.)*. These particular scoring systems merit more detailed explanation:

The Glasgow Coma Scale is the most widely used scoring system for quantifying level of consciousness following traumatic brain injury. Its advantages include the fact that it is simple and easy to use, has a high degree of inter-observer reliability and it correlates well with clinical outcomes. A chart similar to the following is used for documenting the scores, both as individual components and as a total score.

Best Eye Response (4)

1. No eye opening.

2. Eye opening to pain.

3. Eye opening to verbal command.

4. Eyes open spontaneously.

Best Verbal Response (5)

1. No verbal response.

2. Incomprehensible sounds.

3. Inappropriate words.

4. Confused.

5. Orientated.

Best Motor Response (6)
1. No motor response.
2. Extension to pain.
3. Flexion to pain.
4. Withdrawal from pain.
5. Localising pain.
6. Obeys commands.

A coma score of 13 or higher correlates with mild brain injury; 9 to 12 with a moderate injury; 8 or less correlates with a severe brain injury.

The Glasgow Coma Scale has limitations:
(i)   Factors which alter the level of consciousness independently of the brain injury e.g. shock, hypoxia, drug and alcohol intoxication and metabolic disturbances will interfere with the above correlation.
(ii)   Spinal cord injury interferes with the motor response.
(iii)   Orbital trauma may interfere with the eye response.
(iv)   Endotracheal intubation interferes with the verbal response.
(v)   Limited applicability to children especially if younger than 3 years.
When the brain injured patient is intubated, the scale expressed in its individual components may be recorded as E2 V intubated M5.

The Revised Trauma Score is one of the commonly used physiologic scores. It uses three specific physiologic parameters: the Glasgow Coma Scale (GCS), Systolic Blood Pressure (SBP) and the Respiratory Rate (RR). Parameters are coded from 0 to 4 according to the physiologic derangement.

GCS	SPB	RR	Coded Value
13-15	>89	10-29	4
9-12	76-89	>29	3
6-8	50-75	6-9	2
4-5	1-49	1-5	1
3	0	0	0

The Revised Trauma Score has two forms depending on its use. When used for field triage, the RTS is determined by adding all coded values (range 0-12). A score of <11 indicates transfer to a trauma centre. The coded version of RTS, on the other hand, uses coded variables (or multiples) for each variable intended for differential weighting. Thus:

RTSc = 0.9368GCSc + 0.2908RRc + 0.7326 SBPc

Values for RTSc range from 0 to 7.8408. A threshold of < 4 is a certain indication for transfer to a trauma centre. The RTSc correlates well with the probability of survival.

The disadvantages of RTSc include the complicated manner of its computation and all the disadvantages of the GCS already mentioned. Probably the substitution of best motor response on its own for the GCS gives equally good predictions of survival. The Acute Physiology and Chronic Health Evaluation (APACHE) is a system for classifying patients in intensive therapy units. The system is based on two components:

(a) The chronic health evaluation, including the effect of concomitant diseases e.g. diabetes mellitus, COAD.

(b) The Acute Physiology Score (APS).

The APS in APACHE I takes into consideration 8 classes with 34 variables which include the major physiologic systems e.g. cardiovascular: heart rate and mean arterial blood pressure; respiratory: respiratory rate and pACO2 etc. The most abnormal data during the first 24 hours are used to compute the score which is the total number of points referable to all the variables.

The APACHE II score is a general measure of disease severity based on current physiologic measurements (APS), age and previous health condition. The number of APS variables is reduced to just 12, restricting the concomitant diseases and deriving coefficients for specific diseases. The score can help in the assessment of patients to determine the level and degree of diagnostic and therapeutic intervention. Its weakness is related to the absence of an anatomic component in the system.

APACHE III includes 17 variables, limits concomitant diseases to those affecting immune function. It also involves disease-specific equations and includes multiple trauma, distinguishing between brain trauma and trauma to other anatomic parts. It also takes potential lead-time bias into consideration. Unfortunately its software has been commercialised and is expensive. This limits its wide adoption.

Choice of a particular scoring system depends on the proposed use, accuracy of the score and the calibrating equation used (goodness of fit). Rigorous comparative studies are scarce to date. Wide application of scoring systems is limited because the variables may be poorly defined, data may be missed, there may be faults with data collection e.g. observer error or variability and when applied to research, there may be lead time bias i.e. the effects of treatment received before the scoring system is applied. Continued research will hopefully improve methodology and the prediction potential of scoring systems.

The Management of Functional Somatic Symptoms

The interaction between the 'psyche' and 'soma' in disease, which will be referred to again in chapter 5, renders diagnosis and management more difficult and also more interesting. A diagnosis of functional somatic syndrome or symptoms, (psychosomatic disease) should not be reached by exclusion of other somatic disorders but by a 'positive' diagnosis. Clinical symptom-complexes such as aerophagy, irritable bowel syndrome, fibromyalgia, tension headache, chronic fatigue, non-ulcer dyspepsia and non-cardiac chest pain may be considered in this category. Another example of this type of interaction is the high correlation between the intensity of post-operative dysphagia following laparoscopic Nissen 'floppy' fundoplication. and the construct of personality. Patients with high expectations for their own health-related abilities (internal control), had less dysphagia than patients who believed that their convalescence depended more on luck, chance or fate (external control) *(Kamolz, T., Bammer, T., Pointner, R.)*. It is also well established that symptoms of achalasia, itself a 'somatic' disease, are made worse by stress and anxiety. In these cases part of the symptomatology may improve independently from the treatment of the achalasia itself.

The fact that 71% of IBS patients respond to hypnotherapy *(Gonsalkorale, W.M. et al.)*, resulting in fewer consultations and necessity for drug treatment, is indicative of the functional nature of this syndrome.

Functional somatic syndromes are often poorly diagnosed and are not without consequence. Multiple factors may be involved in varying proportions. These include psychological factors e.g. anxiety and depression, biological factors e.g. disturbances of neuronal biochemistry, social factors e.g. marital problems and medico-social factors e.g. litigation *(Mayou, R., Farmer, A.)*. These patients are often psychologically or biologically predisposed e.g. tendency to depression or anxiety and then some precipitating factor e.g. trauma, serious illness in a relative or a friend, bring the symptomatology to the surface. Other factors, such as misdiagnosis, over-investigation, questionable self-directed therapies, occupational stress and the possibility of compensation may perpetuate the symptoms and render them chronic.

The Biological and Psychological Influences on Functional Somatic Disorders:

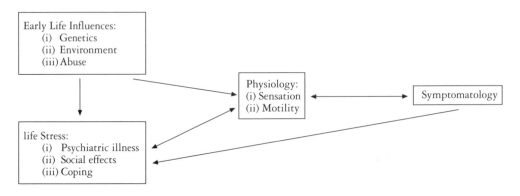

This intricate interaction between what is somatic and what is psychological should discourage the clinician from indulging in an insistent analytical separation of these, but rather concentrate on what can be effectively done to help. One should suspect the possibility of functional somatic symptoms when the symptom complex does not fit into clear-cut pathological or physiological mechanisms, when the symptoms are multiple, varied and unconnected, there are voluminous case notes, indicative observations by medical and paramedical staff and information gathered from relatives. Such information, synthetically but accurately documented, is crucial in clinching the diagnosis and indicating the relative management. Disappearance of the symptoms following such treatment is reassuring, though by no means an absolute proof of the correctness of the diagnosis or management. Patients' symptoms occasionally improve in spite and not because of treatment. Despite all these difficulties, it is most important to detect functional somatic symptoms promptly for several reasons: Untreated anxiety and depression will inhibit response to conventional therapy directed towards the target organs. If not tackled adequately these patients often become 'chronic clinic attendees'. As noted earlier, over-investigation of these cases may well aggravate symptoms. On the other hand, if detected in time, functional somatic syndromes related to organic disease or its treatment e.g. functional somatic symptoms following laparoscopic fundoplication, can be tackled before they result in unnecessary distress.

Most cases presenting with functional somatic symptoms are best managed in primary care and the importance of context effects in this respect cannot be overstressed. One has to explain to the patient that the symptoms are real and not imaginary. The patient should feel confident that he is not being labelled a nut. He will be more receptive if one explains how the biochemical and psychological factors, combined with the precipitating and perpetuating factors active in the particular case may produce their somatic symptoms. The patient may subsequently volunteer further suppressed information. In this atmosphere of mutual confidence it is easier to discuss treatment of any underlying condition and subsequent follow-up.

Effects of Context on Medical Care

Bedside manners, warm patient-doctor relationship and other features of good doctoring contribute to the outcome of medical care (Refer to the second quotation from Hippocrates at the beginning of this chapter). This is illustrated by the results of research on the treatment of diffuse oesophageal spasm: Dilatation with a No. 24 bougie (a dilator of an insignificant calibre), had the same effect as dilatation with a No.50 bougie in improving pain and dysphagia *(Bennett, J.)*. This effect is more obvious in situations rich in personal touch and low in technology such as general practice. Context effects may be small, but can be clinically relevant especially where the efficacy of established therapies is low. The effects may be due to psycho-neuro-immunological responses, or else psychological modifications e.g. raised expectations or conditioned responses. These non-specific effects are integrated into the overall therapeutic process and this relationship merits more research attention. When one considers the preponderance of funding and effort involved in evolving diagnostic and therapeutic innovations, one cannot help feeling that not enough is being done to investigate and put to fruitful use the obvious interaction between psyche and soma which underlie context effects. These frequently manifest themselves as symptoms and disease, are inexpensive when used therpautically and have clear implications on clinical management. These considerations should lead to development of this aspect of therapy and its further weighting in medical curricula and training *(Van Weel, C.).*

The Management of Patients with Chronic Diseases

The planning of care in these cases requires an analysis of the special requirements of patients with chronic diseases. Apart from having to deal with their disabilities, these patients have to deal with the social and psychological impact of their symptoms, as well as the problems of approaching death. They have to take their medicines, interact with available medical care over an increasingly difficult period to alter their way of life and behaviour. The institutions must help this category of patients by providing adequate information, offer the best possible treatment to investigate and control symptoms, provide support for self-management of health and assurance of support after death. The public must be made aware of these problems, which may result in a greater involvement and understanding by the luckier sections of society.

Waiting Lists

The mechanisms which influence waiting lists are poorly understood. Recent evidence indicates that they are mainly influenced by composite local problems and cannot be explained by global disparity in demand and supply, or corrected simply by global funding *(Martin, R.M. et al.).* 25% of U.K. hospital trusts contribute between 50% to 80% of waiting lists extending beyond six months.

Undue waiting lists or 'delays in access to care' may result in:
(i)   Patient and staff dissatisfaction.
(ii) Worsening of clinical outcomes.
(iii) Wasted theatre time because of greater number of patients failing to turn up for surgical procedures.
(iv) Development of complications, which are more difficult and costly to treat *(Murray, M.).*

Streaming cases into urgent and routine queues, does not really help. The more time is allotted to the urgent cases, the less remains for the routine ones. The solution to the problem of waiting lists is to determine the true input and backlog and generate the resources to reduce the latter and deal effectively with the former. Separating elective from emergency surgery could contribute to reduce waiting lists. On the other hand, the distinction between urgent and routine is best eliminated, making sure the lists are kept within reasonable limits. This also involves proper planning for fluctuations in input (e.g. seasonal variations) and supply (e.g. staff vacation leave and refurbishing of operating theatres and wards). Bottlenecks in the delivery of service should be identified and streamlined e.g. the specialist should concentrate on performing the work that makes him unique in the hospital set-up. Other work is delegated, perhaps using guidelines and algorithms.

Waiting lists can be shortened and access made easier by improving the capacity and/or the flexibility of the system, thereby matching or reducing an accurately predicted demand and predictable fluctuations in this demand. In synthesis, the recommended methods to achieve this are those that:

(i)   Gain capacity.
(ii)   Clear backlog.
(iii)   Reduce differential queues or types of visits.
(iv)   Predict and manage fluctuations.
(v)   Reduce demand by encouraging and helping to improve the efficiency of primary care and clearly delineate the boundaries of responsibility for care.
(vi)   Reduce the time wasted by specialists doing things which are not within the confines of their speciality, so that the can concentrate on their 'unique' abilities.
(vii)   Match demand and supply.

The application of operational research, using tools like mathematical modelling, queuing theory and simulation, may help to improve performance. These methods were successfully employed in Alaska *(Murray, M.)*. Containment of waiting lists within reasonable limits actually makes the planning of operating programmes and the management of surgical units less problematic.

Physician Assistants, Nurse Practitioners and Nurse-led Clinics

These categories could constitute one of the ways to tackle the waiting list problem. Physician Assistants and Nurse Practitioners function in similar roles in that both these categories can diagnose, treat and prescribe. As with all other reforms these have advantages and disadvantages:

Physician Assistants	Nurse Practitioners	Nurse-led Clinics
Training is generalist in nature, based on medical school rotations and curricula.	Speciality based	Nurses trained to perform specialized tasks as part of a team under the overall responsibility of a consultant.
Medical background and set-up	Nursing background – a form of advanced nursing practice.	Advantages: (i) Allows continuity of care more than can be achieved with rotating junior medical staff. (ii) Medical staff have more time for other clinical duties. (iii) Economic considerations.
	2 key areas of application: (i) as members of primary health care teams. (ii) specialised care of specific groups. (Lenehan C)	Disadvantages: (i) Medico-legal consequences of delegation. (ii) Medical junior staff may loose out on experience *(Murray WJG)*.

Patients' Reaction to Surgery

People attribute a meaning to all events in life and this includes surgical procedures. This meaning depends on a number of variables and will eventually result in an emotional response, which will eventually induce physiological changes, distinct and additive to the better-documented physiological response to surgical trauma. This psychologically mediated physiological response is at least partly mediated by the hypothalamo-pituitary-adrenal axis and the autonomic nervous system *(Petry, J.)*.

Traditionally doctors tend to attenuate these adverse effects by prescribing pharmacological sedation. This has the advantage of being simple and having immediate effect, but unfortunately this effect tends to be very transient. The literature provides countless alternative methods, some little more than quackery, which presumably give the same or better results. Actually, the most practical and useful method is dialogue. This enhances the doctor - patient relationship and explores the individual meaning that the intended surgical procedure has for the patient. It helps the patient to deal with the fears, worries and prejudices, as well as to correct any misconceptions. This method is only costly in terms of time. However it pays back handsomely as regards benefit to the patient and often to the surgeon Apart from psychologically mediated response, the peripheral and central nervous system is crucial in initiating the endocrine metabolic response to trauma. Regional anaesthesia can reduce this response, improving postoperative catabolism and glucose intolerance, while it does not modify inflammatory or immunological response. Generally this results in a 30% reduction in morbidity compared with general anaesthesia with proper selection of cases *(Rodgers, A. et al.)*. Maintenance of normal patient temperature is another factor, which reduces the stress of surgical procedures. Patients should be given adequate and timely instructions regarding cessation of smoking 1 – 2 months pre-operatively, abstinence from alcohol and proper control of chronic debilities e.g. diabetes. Not only does this contribute to reduce morbidity and mortality, but it also allows wider use of fast track surgery.

To elaborate further on the value of pre-operative abstinence from smoking the following is a synopsis of the evidence:

1. Stopping smoking for 12 hours pre-operatively prevents the adverse effects of carbon monoxide and nicotine on myocardial oxygen supply and demand *(Nel MR, Morgan, M.)*.
2. Stopping smoking for a few days improves ciliary action *(Egan, T.D., Wong, K.C.)*.
3. Abstinence from smoking for 6 weeks reduces the post-operative pulmonary complications, which are 2 to 6 times more frequent in smokers *(Jones, R.M., Rosen, M., Seymour, L.)*.
4. Stopping for 8 weeks reduces the mortality to the levels of non-smokers in patients undergoing CABG *(Warner, M.A. et al.)*.
5. Passive smoking increases post-operative pulmonary complications in children *(Skolnick, E.T. et al.)*. This probably also applies to adults.
6. Smokers also have an increased incidence of surgical complications resulting in direct and indirect vascular damage and impaired wound healing from tissue hypoxia ant smoke toxins *(Kripski, W.C.)*.

Prophylaxis

Prophylactic therapies are meant to prevent the development of serious disease. These may take the form of vaccines, prophylactic medical therapy, such as prophylactic antibiotic regimens, which will be discussed later on in this chapter and even prophylactic surgery.

The development of vaccines is one of the most important advances in medicine, providing populations with the necessary immunological tools against infectious agents. They may be directed against micro organisms e.g. conjugated pneumococcal vaccine, toxins e.g. tetanus toxoid, and even non-infectious diseases e.g. diabetes, Alzheimer's disease, certain types of cancer and even drug dependence. Easier delivery routes than the traditional parenteral route, e.g. nasal, oral, trans-cutaneous and depot preparations are being developed.

Prophylactic surgical procedures are only carried out on persons at risk. The advances in molecular genetics will, most likely, widen the indications for this aspect of therapy, which includes proctocolectomy for ulcerative colitis, Crohn's colits and familial polyposis coli, prophylactic mastectomy in the contralateral breast in breast cancer cases and in persons at high risk of developing this disease.

Surgical Treatment - Introduction

It may be considered anachronistic that we are discussing treatment in surgery when we have been talking of 'surgical management' in the previous sections. This is being done out of convenience, well knowing that in the management of the surgical patient, treatment may not necessarily follow the establishment of a definite diagnosis chronologically.

SURGERY

Furthermore, surgical treatment can hardly be learned from a book or lecture - no cookery book ever made a chef! Such a practical subject must be studied at the bedside and in the operating theatre, with personal guidance from a senior colleague. This apprenticeship method involves graded exposure to surgical technique based on the trainee's progress. Because this method is time-consuming, it may clash with the move towards shorter working hours for trainees, the self-interest of the teacher and the economic constraints of the institution. This has encouraged the adoption of different modalities for training, which is directed towards component operative generic skills performed in special skills laboratories e.g. suturing, anastomotic techniques and laparoscopic skills. Research on outcomes from this change in emphasis is to be encouraged.

Cuschieri surgical skills unit (Ninewells)

The value of many current treatments remains obscure, since these have never been scientifically assessed. One investigation reported that five of the ten most commonly performed operations in the U.K. had no proven benefit *(Towle, A.)*. Most prophylactic treatments, if at all effective, have only a modest impact on overall morbidity and mortality. This may seem to be unkind on the medical profession and calls for analysis of sources, subject, method etc. of this study. However, any variation in the conclusions, as a result of such analysis, may only be one of degree or proportion. It is a fact that many new procedures are adopted without formal ethical or scientific scrutiny and are judged by their early results, even if they are meant to have long-term effects.

Furthermore, the method of action of a significant proportion of present therapies is poorly or incompletely understood. Successful outcome does not necessarily mean that this was the result of the treatment, even if, basing on present knowledge, the administration of a therapy may seem logical. The removal of impurities from the body by venisection and the use of leeches is an example from the past, which surely has modern analogies. The use of HRT to reduce the incidence of myocardial infarction and the routine use of pre-operative blood investigations are examples of ineffective procedures in current use. If we do not succeed in pruning these and similar useless or harmful treatments, it will be for future generations to rectify them. On the other hand, incomplete knowledge of the modus operandi of a therapy does not necessarily mean that the treatment is ineffective. For example, we are still ignorant as to whether probiotics such as lactobacilli or bifidobacteria prevent antibiotic induced diarrhoea by occupying binding sites on the gut mucosa at the expense of pathogens, by producing local antibiotics against these, by competing with pathogens for nutrients, by strengthening the T helper 1 cells concerned with immune response and reducing the T helper 2 cell allergic response or by some

Q Discovery Drugs

other method. Meta-analysis of several reliable trials shows that probiotics are effective and their low cost and rarity of side effects may make them an attractive therapeutic option despite our ignorance of their mode of action.

When the benefits of a new therapy are uncertain, one can only carefully evaluate existing evidence. Even this may be insufficient to eliminate the uncertainty. Health authorities should formally record and review these known 'uncertainties' and this information should be made available to clinicians. This would enable clinicians to discuss these uncertainties with their patients, being well aware that such disclosures may undermine the patient's confidence in his doctor. A general debate amongst all concerned is however appropriate.

One must resist the blind following of rituals, the compulsion to act at all costs and to feel constrained to satisfy patients' expectations regardless. One must also be suspicious of surrogate outcomes and treatments based only on empiricism.

Ideally a doctor owes his patient all the resources of his science (refer to statement 6 of the Hippocratic Oath). Resources are, however, limited and demands are increasing as a result of an ageing population, emphasis on quality and choice, and new technologies often with (perhaps artificially) inflated prices. Thus this ethical consideration cannot be applied uncritically. Only the patient has a right to deny himself a universally accepted and available treatment, but not the right to demand a treatment that cannot be offered to others in the same position as well. Because of the ageing population, and since most of our lifetime health expenditure occurs during old age, there is a strong financial incentive to develop expensive treatments directed at the older age group. This is far more profitable, for the medical companies than preventive measures. The resulting soaring costs of health schemes are difficult to sustain by many countries. Medical students should be made aware of this, through their medical curricula. Furthermore, The attitude of potent governments when confronting the dilemma of drug patents in the face of public health emergencies has been blatantly double-faced. This is evidenced by the contrasting attitudes towards the treatment of the HIV positive in developing countries and anthrax therapy in the US and Canada.

One has to identify efficient treatments and implement them through practice guidelines, policies (e.g. Antibiotic Policy), protocols and computerised decision support systems. One example is the application of protocols for antibiotic prophylaxis in 'clean-contaminated' surgical wounds, which results in a markedly reduced wound infection rate and real cost benefit. Even where such aids to patient management are applicable, there is a serious staffing problem in most countries, which is an impediment to the achievement of the above- mentioned ideals. The reasons for this shortage include: an accelerated trend towards early retirement amongst consultants (at present, the average retiring age of consultant surgeons in UK is 57 years), increased need for consultants with the shift from a consultant-led to a consultant-delivered system, higher proportion of female doctors than in the past (these often end up working on a less than full time basis), the increasing proportion of emergency to elective hospital admissions and the development of the private health sector. On the nursing side, poor pay and conditions, illogical distribution of manpower and, to some extent, the institution of the nursing degree have hindered recruitment and induced a drain. It is to be expected that the adoption of the European directives on mutual recognition of specialist qualifications, the trend towards hyperspecialisation and the pressure by medical and nursing associations and unions, may complicate the staffing situation even further. These problems in the delivery of health care are an incentive to make a concerted effort to make best use of available resources, whilst admitting our limitations, at any particular time.

Decision making in Surgical Treatment

When making decisions about treatment, surgical or medical, one should

(i)   Identify the ultimate objective of treatment e.g. cure, palliation, symptomatic relief, prevention of complications etc.
(ii)   Select the best treatment taking all available data in consideration.
(iii)   Specify treatment target, so as to know when to stop or change treatment etc.

The practical nature of surgical treatment calls for concrete examples. I shall here attempt to illustrate general principles in treatment with reference to four particular surgical situations:

A. Antibiotics in the treatment of surgical infections,

B. The acute abdomen,

C. Acute scrotal pain,

D. Intravenous fluid regimens in cases of peritonitis in infants.

One may object that the situations to be discussed are 'simple and straightforward ones' whereas this cannot be said of many other clinical conditions. Though this is in part a valid point, one has to recognise that delineating methods for solving 'simple and straightforward' clinical problems, will help us in unravelling more complex ones. It is in the very nature of examples to be simple and clear.

A.   Antibiotics in the Treatment of Surgical Infections

Sepsis is still an important cause of morbidity and death in our patients. The awareness of the limitation of antibiotics and the need of defining their role has stimulated a multitude of trials and publications of varying quality. Actually, the prophylaxis and treatment of sepsis should be based on six cornerstones:

(i)   strict observation of aseptic technique,
(ii)   proper surgical technique,
(iii)   adequate drainage where indicated,
(iv)   correct use of antibiotics in prophylaxis and treatment of infection.
(v)   hygiene,
(vi)   vaccines.
(Felice, Cuschieri, Caruana Montalto, Zarb Adami, Cacciottolo).

In the choice of antibiotics three factors are of paramount importance:

(a)   the pharmacokinetic properties of the antibiotic,
(b)   its toxicity,
(c)   its anti microbial spectrum and frequency of antibiotic resistance.

Thus, to be able to reach all types of infections, an antibiotic must have a low degree of toxicity to allow for the use of very high doses when infections at sites which are difficult to penetrate are treated, and kinetic properties which readily enable them to pass into deep (poorly accessible) compartments. In addition, it must be active, where necessary, against several bacterial species in the clinical situation, which is often less favourable for antibacterial activity, than in vitro techniques indicate.

These pharmacokinetic properties involve the following factors:

(i)   Gastro-intestinal absorption - it determines plasma and tissue levels,

(ii)   Protein binding - only the free (unbound) fraction of the antibiotics is able to penetrate a peripheral compartment if it is not lipid soluble. This is of practical importance if protein binding is more than 80%,

(iii)   Lipid solubility - this facilitates the penetration of an antibiotic into a peripheral compartment,

(iv)   Metabolism - if an antibiotic is metabolised, most metabolites have a lower antimicrobial effect than their parent compound,

(v)   Elimination - antibiotics are eliminated either via the kidneys by glomerular filtration and/or tubular secretion, or via hepatic metabolism and/or biliary excretion. This knowledge is necessary in choosing the antibiotic for specific problems e.g. Urinary tract or biliary tract infections, and for correcting doses in cases of reduced hepatic or renal function,

(vi) Tissue penetration - what is important is the concentration of free (active) drug in peripheral compartments except in cases of septicaemia.

Compartments are usually classified as:

(a) Shallow compartments, e.g. peritoneal, pleural, pericardial and interstitial fluids. Here antibiotic concentrations parallel serum concentrations. Protein binding carries less weight and most antibiotics can be used therapeutically and prophylactically.

(b) Moderately deep compartments, e.g. infections with fibrin deposition but no abscess formation, saliva, the middle ear and maxillary sinuses. Peak concentrations here occur within 30 minutes of i.v. administration.

(c) Deep compartments - where there is hindrance of passive diffusion or the volume of the compartment is large, e.g. blood-brain barrier due to non-fenestrated capillaries and blood-CSF barrier due to tight junctions in the choroid plexus, and abscesses. Peak concentrations are lower than in plasma and occur about an hour after an i.v. dose. On the other hand, elimination is likewise slower and accumulation can occur *(Ragnor Norrby, S.)*.

Guidelines on antibiotic regimes have been drawn up keeping the above factors in mind (vide. Antibiotic Policy) but they should not be regarded as single modality treatment of any infection *(Felice, A. et al.)*.

Micro-organisms show great ingenuity in blocking the effects of antimicrobial agents with the development of antibiotic resistance e.g. MRSA, vancomycin resistant MRSA, penicillin resistant pneumococci, etc. Since bacteria may double their number every 20 minutes, resistant mutants have a great selective advantage in the presence of antibiotics. Unfortunately antibiotics are all too frequently misused in human and veterinary medicine, farming (growth promoters), aqua culture and plant culture. When antibiotics are administered to humans, the normal bacterial flora in the body are also exposed to the drug, and since most antibiotics are excreted in the active form, environmental bacteria are also exposed (hence the problems encountered in water recycling plants from sewage).

Antibiotic resistant genes existed well before antibiotics were used – resistant bacteria have been grown from 2000 years old deep ice in the Arctic. The worrying aspect is that antibiotic resistant genes may be transferred both vertically down generations of bacteria and horizontally to other bacteria, species and genera by means of plasmids. Furthermore, these can accumulate different resistance genes (integrons and transposons) sequentially forming large plasmids encoding multidrug resistance *(Hart, C.A.)*.

There are several incorrect motions and myths relating to bacterial antibiotic resistance:

1. Antibiotic resistance is inevitable if an antibiotic is used in sufficient volume over time. This is incorrect. Doxycycline and nitrofurantoin have been used in considerable volumes over decades without the emergence of significant resistance. Experience with limiting the use of sulphonamides nationwide did not result in decrease of sulphonamide-resistant E. coli.
2. Antibiotic resistance is related to certain antibiotic classes e.g. 3rd generation cephalosporins and fluoroquinolonnes. This is also incorrect. Resistance varies greatly within the classes e.g. antibiotic resistance to Ceftazidime but not to other 3rd generation cephalosporins; to gentamycin but not to amicacin; to imipenem but not to meropenem.
3. Clonal resistance is perpetuated by inappropriate antibiotic use. Again this is incorrect. Clonal resistance is spread and perpetuated by ineffective infection control measures *(Cunha, B.A.)*.

   It is important to understand the concept of 'Antibiotic – resistance – potential': If resistance develops during drug development, during clinical trials or within two years of general use, the antibiotic is categorized as having high-resistance–potential.

   Beyond this time antibiotic resistance rarely develops. In this latter category, antibiotics are considered as having low-resistance-potential. The chances are that they will be used freely for decades without fear of emergence of resistant strains.

In an attempt to avoid defeat in the antibiotic war with resistant strains, one should:

(i) Educate doctors, veterinary surgeons, horticulturists and the public on correct use of antimicrobials including regular publishing of antibiotic policy.

(ii) Apply more emphasis on this subject in the undergraduate curriculum.

(iii) Develop surveillance systems for antimicrobial resistance.

(iv) The use of antibiotics in veterinary and horticultural fields, which antibiotics are also used in human disease, should be dealt with great consideration and care, as well as under strict control. More specifically the addition of antibiotics to animal feeds and products should be banned, considering the large volumes used and the inevitability that these will eventually affect humans.

(v) Restrict access and use of antibiotics with high resistance potential. This should be emphasised in antibiotic policies and formularies.

(vi) Preferably use antibiotics with low resistance potential.

(vii) Take measures to contain highly resistant clones within the hospital environment.

(viii) Not apply the concept of antibiotic cycling if antibiotics with high resistance potential are used.

(ix) If a particular resistance problem is shown to be due to a single agent, then simple substitution is logical. In case of multiple resistance, the restriction of other high – resistance – potential antibiotics is mandatory. As an example, when one comes across penicillin resistant pneumococci, macrolides co-trimoxazole and ciprofloxacin may have to be restricted.

(x) More resources should be directed to research on antimicrobial resistance.

B. *Treatment of the Acute Abdomen*

The 'Acute abdominal situation' refers to abdominal symptoms, which have lasted less than eight days and suggest a disease which definitely or possibly threatens life (*Jones, P.F.*). This may result from:

(a) Obstruction of a hollow viscus,
(b) Peritoneal irritation due to inflammation, ischaemia or perforation of an abdominal organ.
(c) Haemorrhage.

The resulting pathophysiology will threaten life due to:

1. Sepsis
2. Acute disturbance of body fluids from
   (i) Blood loss
   (ii) Plasma loss
   (iii) Fluid and electrolyte disturbance.

The treatment administered to the patient should be directed at:

(a) correcting the pathophysiology described above,
(b) correcting or removing the cause.

The avenues for management of these conditions are not all available to the various clinicians that are confronted with the problem.

As an example, the **General Practitioner** outside hospital facing a patient with a possible acute abdomen is mainly concerned with the selection of patients, which need hospital referral. The following scheme attempts to illustrate guidelines for this purpose:

Chart 4.1 – *Hospital referral*

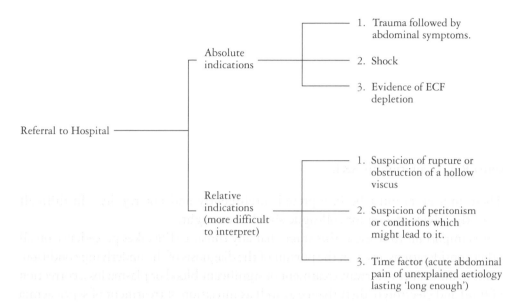

The **Casualty Officer's** role in management is to administer emergency treatment to deal with the immediate life threatening situation, to request the necessary urgent investigations and to select and pigeon-hole the patients referred to the A&E Department. The possible avenues are illustrated below:

Chart 4.2 – *Patient referral*

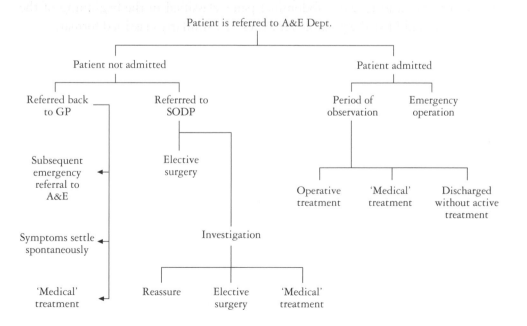

There is no substitute to clinical acumen in guiding the Casualty Officer in his decisions though one could provide lists of indications for, (or risk factors indicating) hospital admission such as follows:

(i)   Pain lasting less than 48 hours,

(ii)   Pain followed by vomiting,

(iii)   Impairment of consciousness,

(iv)   History of recent trauma, operation or haemorrhage,

(v)   Abnormal physical signs,

(vii) Sometimes extremes of age,

(viii) Representation to A&E.

These indicators must be interpreted intelligently and not rigidly. In difficult cases the advice of a senior colleague should be sought.

It is important to stress at this stage that any threat to life takes precedence on all other considerations, even on the pursuit of the diagnosis of the underlying condition. Thus maintenance of airway, treatment of significant blood or plasma loss, correction of fluid and electrolyte disturbance as well as initiation of treatment of septicaemia takes priority over other aspects of management.

The **Surgical Team** then is responsible for continuing or altering the treatment initiated in the A&E Department, depending on the clinical situation. The causative pathology has then to be dealt with.

It is not the purpose of this discussion to go into the details of treatment of the various aetiologies of the acute abdomen. Referring back to the broad pathological causes that may lead to acute abdominal pains classified in the beginning of the chapter, one could list the possible remedies in a similarly classified format:

Chart 4.3 *–Treatment of obstruction of a hollow viscus*

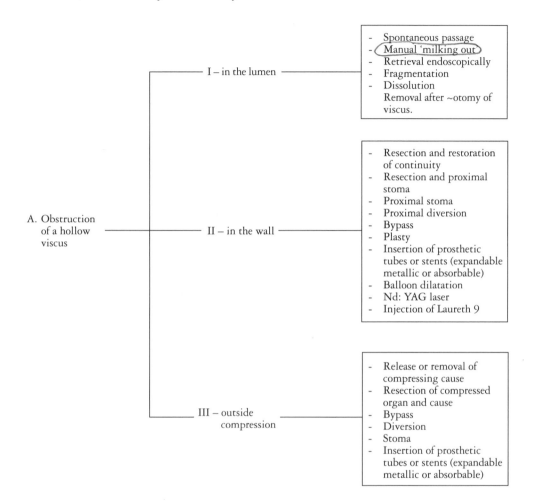

Chart 4.4 *–Treatment of peritoneal irritation*

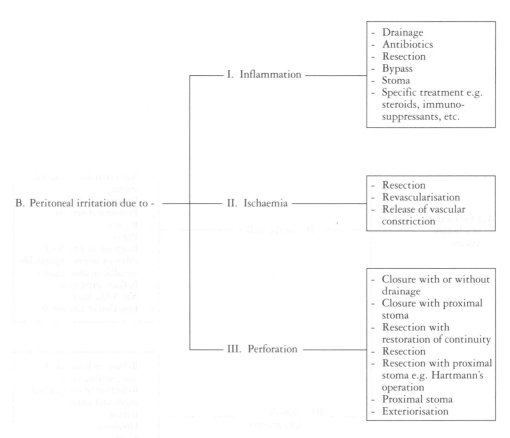

Chart 4.5 *–Treatment of Haemorrhage*

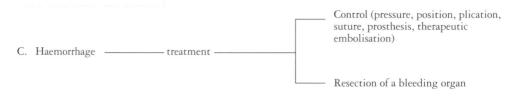

This is an attempt to illustrate a logical approach to a very complex and difficult clinical problem at the cost of possible oversimplification. The techniques range from pharmacological, to laparoscopy, to formal laparotomy.

Algorithms may be helpful in serving as guidelines in this hazardous terrain. Examples of these are reproduced from the paper on the subject by *Martin, R.F.* and *Rossi, R.L.* in the Surgical Clinics of North America as depicted by charts 4.6 to 4.9. One should note that charts 4.8 and 4.9 are not really algorithms but lists for differential diagnosis as an adjunct to the algorithms in charts 4.6 and 4.7.

Chart 4.6 *–Treatment of Acute Abdominal Pain*

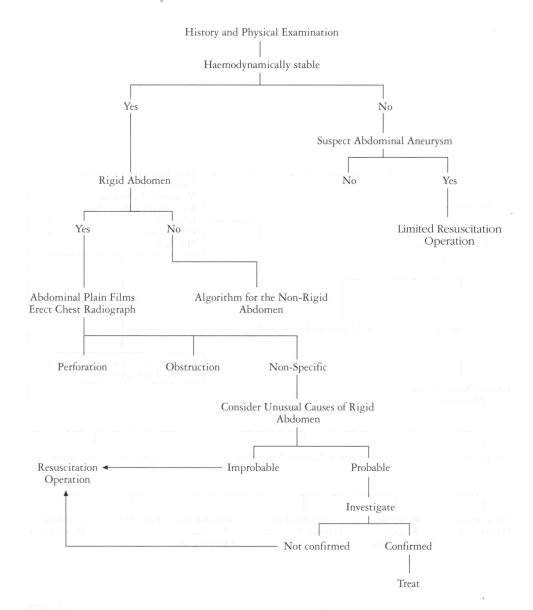

(1997)

Chart 4.7 – *The Non-Rigid Abdomen*

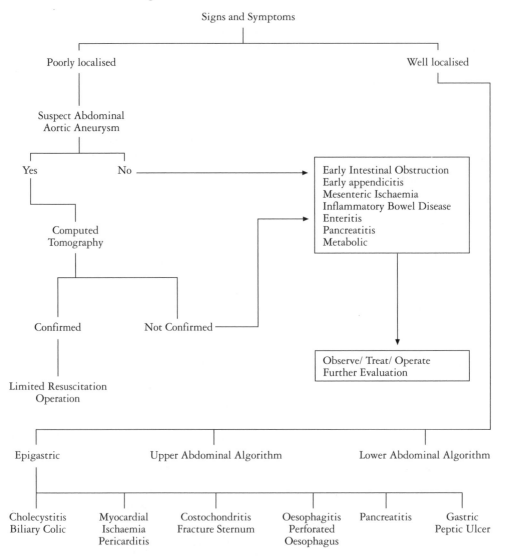

(1997)

Chart 4.8 – *Upper Abdominal Pain:*

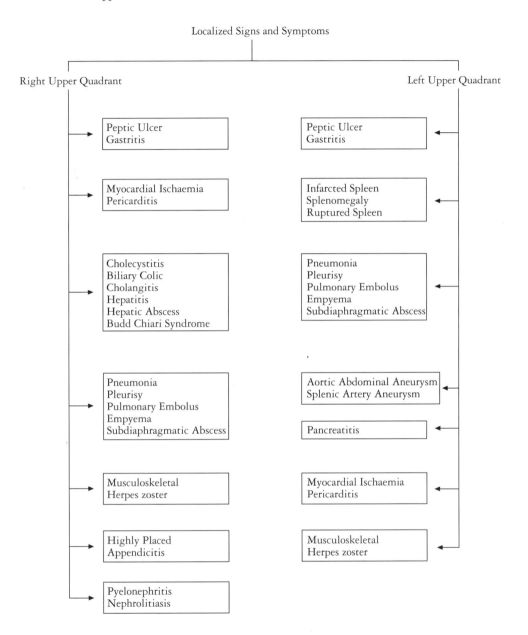

Localized Signs and Symptoms

Right Upper Quadrant   Left Upper Quadrant

| Peptic Ulcer |
| Gastritis |

| Peptic Ulcer |
| Gastritis |

| Myocardial Ischaemia |
| Pericarditis |

| Infarcted Spleen |
| Splenomegaly |
| Ruptured Spleen |

| Cholecystitis |
| Biliary Colic |
| Cholangitis |
| Hepatitis |
| Hepatic Abscess |
| Budd Chiari Syndrome |

| Pneumonia |
| Pleurisy |
| Pulmonary Embolus |
| Empyema |
| Subdiaphragmatic Abscess |

| Pneumonia |
| Pleurisy |
| Pulmonary Embolus |
| Empyema |
| Subdiaphragmatic Abscess |

| Aortic Abdominal Aneurysm |
| Splenic Artery Aneurysm |

| Pancreatitis |

| Musculoskeletal |
| Herpes zoster |

| Myocardial Ischaemia |
| Pericarditis |

| Highly Placed |
| Appendicitis |

| Musculoskeletal |
| Herpes zoster |

| Pyelonephritis |
| Nephrolitiasis |

(1997)

Chart 4.9 – *Lower Abdominal Pain:*

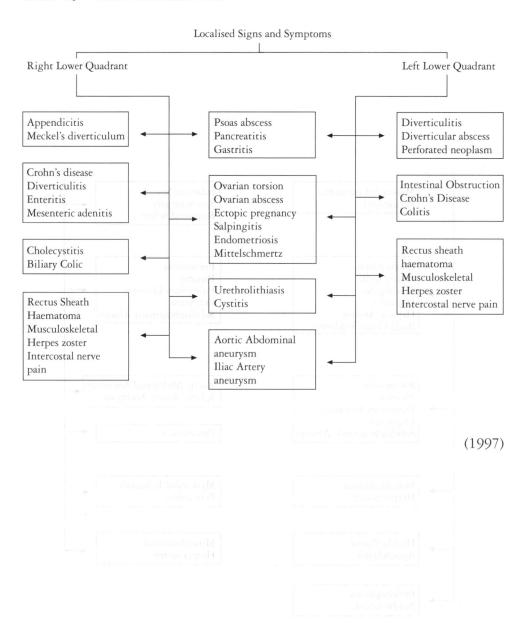

Localised Signs and Symptoms

Right Lower Quadrant

Left Lower Quadrant

Appendicitis
Meckel's diverticulum

Psoas abscess
Pancreatitis
Gastritis

Diverticulitis
Diverticular abscess
Perforated neoplasm

Crohn's disease
Diverticulitis
Enteritis
Mesenteric adenitis

Ovarian torsion
Ovarian abscess
Ectopic pregnancy
Salpingitis
Endometriosis
Mittelschmertz

Intestinal Obstruction
Crohn's Disease
Colitis

Cholecystitis
Biliary Colic

Rectus sheath
haematoma
Musculoskeletal
Herpes zoster
Intercostal nerve pain

Rectus Sheath
Haematoma
Musculoskeletal
Herpes zoster
Intercostal nerve
pain

Urethrolithiasis
Cystitis

Aortic Abdominal
aneurysm
Iliac Artery
aneurysm

(1997)

Chart 4.10 – *Right Lower Quadrant Pain:*

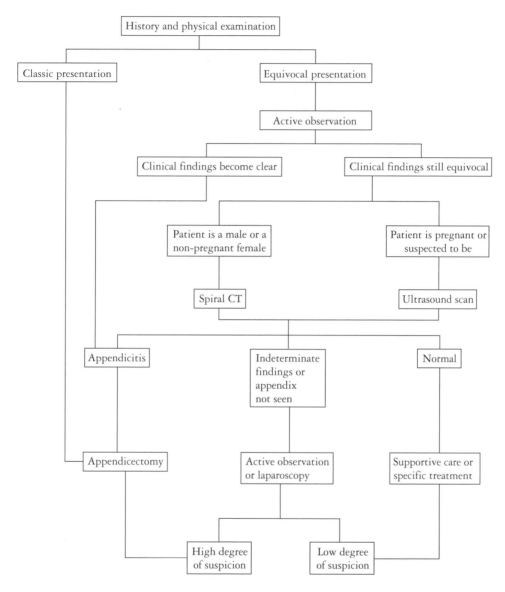

C. Acute Scrotal Pain

When one is planning the treatment of a case presenting with acute scrotal pain, one must consider the possible causes as well as the consequences of the pathology and of the treatment being planned.

The possible causes are:

(i) torsion of the spermatic cord (of the testicles),

(ii) torsion of an appendage of the testicle (hydatid of Morgagni),

(iii) acute epididymo-orchitis,

(iv) acute orchitis (mumps, Henoch-Schonlein purpura),

(v) trauma.

Because of the tragic consequences of missing a torsion of the spermatic cord (delaying operation by 12-18 hours causes testicular infarction), it should be an absolute rule to explore all cases presenting with acute scrotal pain where one cannot clearly make out the epididymis to be inflamed and distinct from the testicle. The use of ultrasound, radioisotope scanning and Doppler of testicular vessels may lead to procrastination delays and increased rate of infarction of the testicles.

If the presumptive diagnosis of torsion of the spermatic cord is confirmed at operation, one untwists the mesorchium (most torsions are intra-vaginal) and inspects the vascularity of the testicle. If the testicle is black, does not bleed and is frankly dead, an orchiectomy is carried out. If the testicle is viable or if there is any doubt as to its viability, it should be returned to the scrotum and fixed by suturing or by creating a dartos pouch. Since the underlying abnormality of the tunica is bilateral, the contralateral testicle is also fixed at the same operation or a few days later. Failure to do this might endanger the patient's fertility.

If at operation one finds some other cause of testicular pain, e.g. torsion of a testicular appendage or haemorrhage from trauma, operative treatment may still be helpful, i.e. excision of torted appendage or control of haemorrhage and evacuation of the blood if the cause is trauma to the testicle.

Even if epididymo-orchitis is found at operation, the surgeon should not feel ashamed even though the first line treatment for this is non-surgical. The operation will serve to ensure diagnosis and enable him to initiate antibiotic therapy. It will also show that he is aware of tragic consequences of missing a torsion of the testicle.

D.   *Intravenous Fluid Regimens in Cases of Peritonitis in Infants*

These regimens are usually based on theoretical considerations, experimentation (in animal and/or human models), and experience with assessment of results.

The administration of intravenous fluids in infants who have developed peritonitis is notoriously difficult and hazardous due to a high surface area to volume ratio and other physiological considerations. Various regimens, using the above-mentioned methods, have been drawn out. The clinician chooses the regimen, which appears to have the best scientific backing and results and then assesses this in his own practice. The results are evaluated and the conclusions of this process will determine whether the regimen will become established in the procedures of the clinician's surgical unit. The particular technique will stand the test of time until a 'possibly better' technique is brought forward, or until flaws or defects in the results of the method, including any inconvenience that may be an intrinsic part of the regimen, becomes apparent.

When one suggests a regimen for i.v. fluids, the first consideration is the type of fluid to be used.   In cases of peritonitis one tries to replace whatever type of fluid and electrolytes are lost during this pathology as accurately as possible. This is usually determined by theoretical considerations and experimentation. In this particular pathology it has been determined that initially the fluids lost are mainly water and electrolytes which are practically identical in concentration to those in the serum. Later on, one looses protein rich exudate into the peritoneal cavity. Thus the fluids used in the treatment of this condition are tailored accordingly and one tends to use Hartmann's solution or 5% Dextrose in $\frac{1}{4}$ strength saline only in cases presenting early, but supplements these with colloid preparations in late cases.

The next consideration is the rate of infusion (i.e. the amount) of fluids needed. These are determined by experimentation initially and subsequently by evaluation of clinical application with monitoring of effects.

One example of such a regimen is as follows:
    Maintenance rate of fluids given is related to the child's mass and surface area:

    up to 10 Kgs   –   100 mls/kg/day
    10 - 20 Kgs   –   50 mls/kg/day
    beyond 20 Kgs   –   20 mls/kg/day with a maximum cut-off at 1.5 litres.

The volume and rate to replace pathological losses has, obviously, to be over and above simple maintenance. One method is to divide the child's abdomen into four imaginary quadrants. One then gives $\frac{1}{4}$ of the maintenance volume for each quadrant affected by the intra-abdominal pathology in addition to the normal maintenance volume infusion over 24 hours. This means that the infusion of fluids should be double the maintenance amount in a case of generalised peritonitis.

Prevention of Disease
The ideal way of managing any disease is by preventing its onset, its progress, or its complications. Preventive medicine thus depends on the natural history of the disease and can be applied at three levels:
a) Primary prevention – aimed at preventing the onset of the health problem, e.g. educating children against smoking or on balanced diets.
b) Secondary prevention – aimed at halting the progression of disease, based on early detection and diagnosis, e.g. cervical screening.
c) Tertiary prevention – aimed at preventing complications or further complications of established disease, e.g. rehabilitation following limb amputations or after myocardial infarction *(Wilson, A.)*.
One health problem which has not been effected by progress in preventive medicine is trauma i.e. injuries or accidents, despite the fact that this is a number one killer

and a cause of serious disability especially in young people and is practically always preventable. Medical counselling and education dose not seem to make a dent in the rate of injuries because it does not alter behaviour sufficiently to produce this result. This contrasts with the effects of medical education against smoking and obesity. Whether this is the effect of insufficient training in such counselling or an intrinsic insufficiency of the method, is not clear. We certainly have to rely on laws and regulations to reduce accident rates.

In general, the focus of health care has shifted from cure of disease to preservation of health, and from individual and episodic to comprehensive and continuous care.

Integrated Care Pathways

These are care plans which detail essential steps in the care of patients with a specific clinical problem and describe the expected clinical course *(Coffey, R.J. et al.)*.

They aim to facilitate the introduction into clinical practice of clinical guidelines and audit as well as aiding communications with patients.

Integrated care pathways are convenient in that they take little writing to complete. They also encourage an multidisciplinary approach to patient care, make data collection more easily available and enable new staff to learn quickly the necessary protocols minimising mistakes.

When problems are complex Integrated Care Pathways are difficult to apply. They may potentially lead the clinician along an 'automatic' prefixed track discouraging personalised management in specific cases or even clear thinking about the clinical problem and therefore may even hinder innovation and progress.

Integrated Care Pathways are just one aspect of the use of protocols (treatment vehicles e.g. Bowel preparation for large bowel surgery, anticoagulation regimens.) and guidelines (aide memoirs in management) and their effectiveness has still to be evaluated *(Campbell, H. et al.)*.

Clinical Networks

These have been defined as 'linked groups of health professionals and organisations from primary, secondary and tertiary care, working in co-ordination, unconstrained by existing professional and organisational boundaries, to ensure equitable provision of high quality medical services'. *(The Scottish Office, Dept. of Health)*. Networks may be subdivided by function, type of disease, specialty or patient group. Their advantages include: more flexibility and rapidity of action focusing on clinical issues, making best use of scarce specialist expertise and faster spread of innovation, fostering creativity and inter-professional communication. On the other hand, their introduction may cause confusion regarding boundaries of responsibility and competence. One hopes they do not end up as another structural change which solves few problems, whilst creating others, and will just form another body in the health service hierarchy.

Iatrogenesis

One usually thinks of iatrogenic harm in terms of clinical iatrogenesis, that is, injury inflicted on patients by ineffective, toxic or unsafe treatments. However iatrogenesis may also have a social form. Through medicalisation, social problems are presented as diseases, turning people inopportunely into patients and consumers of medicine. People may also be harmed through cultural iatrogenesis by destroying the traditional ways of looking at, and dealing with, inevitable death, pain and suffering *(Illich, I.)*.

Clinical Risk Management

Though the development of these strategies was prompted by pressures from medical negligence litigation, these should be regarded as attempts to improve the quality of care and reduce the incidence of harm done to patients. They are not simply attempts to reduce compensation costs. When one considers that about 16.6% of hospital admissions result in adverse effects, of which half were considered preventable *(Wilson, R.M. et al.)*, and the high cost of this to patients, hospitals and the state, one has to admit that these strategies are justified. If one defines adverse events as injuries caused by medical management that prolongs hospitalisation or produces disability at the time of discharge, then the figure comes down to a more realistic 4% (or slightly less then this). Mistakes and near misses should be investigated and analysed in a positive way, leading to practical and specific suggestions as to how to avoid these mishaps and how to effectively deal with them when they occur. It is in the patients' best interest and also in our own, to develop better systems to deal with error.

Litigation

Reports and advice from medical defence organizations are most instructive in that they warn that certain procedures may lead to litigation and unfavourable judgements.

When is a claim for compensation justified? A patient who proves that a condition from which he is suffering is a probable consequence of medical treatment or the withholding of this, can rightfully claim for compensation unless:

a. The complaint is a consequence of the patient's original disease or condition.
b. Is an inevitable, foreseeable or predictable consequence of the treatment, about which the patient was adequately informed.
c. The ageing process.

   Defence against a compensation claim would be base on these three exceptions. The relevant authorities have to set rules for procedures for compensation claims and for the levels of such claims. Clinical negligence claims are invariably settled on the evidence of ones own peers, who report on the adequacy of one's practice.

It is anachronistic that society considers it fit to compensate adverse effects resulting from clinical events, but not other adverse results, which include congenital abnormalities and 'acts of God'. This is hardly fair or even logical but is justified by the limitation of resources. Society considers that it would be far too costly to be fair!

Medical Technology

We have seen that the sequence of actions in clinical practice can, most often, be illustrated as:

History taking and physical examination, selection of diagnostic tests, evaluation of diagnostic tests, diagnostic flow chart or correlation with known pathology, diagnosis, selection of treatment modalities, treatment, monitoring of treatment and evaluation of results *(Anbar, M.)*.

There is no step in this sequence, which does not depend on technology and this dependence is bound to become more pronounced. The introduction of new technologies often allows us to be more quantitative and objective in our clinical assessment than was previously possible, and this is sometimes crucial in difficult clinical or operative situations involving close-call decisions. An example is provided by the intra-operative assessment of intestinal viability following strangulation. This is usually assessed on the basis of crude observations e.g. intestinal colour, peristalsis, arterial pulsations or bleeding from pinprick. All these involve subjective interpretation. New technologies allow a more objective assessment: Using a charge-couple device microscope one can measure the velocity of blood cells in fourth order venules in a doubtful intestinal segment intra-operatively and this is compared with that in a reference segment. A ratio >0.76 is associated with a favourable outcome. Another helpful technology is the U.S. National Institute of Health Imaging, which shows the ratio of area of effective functioning vessels. A ratio >0.54 is associated with a good prognosis *(Yasumura, M. et al.)*.

Descriptive research has shown that diffusion of any technology, including new methods of medical or surgical therapy, follows a sigmoid curve: The early phase of diffusion is slow, reflecting caution on the part of the users and difficulties in communication. Acceptance increases when the technology is shown to be beneficial. Eventually, when most potential adopters of the innovation have accepted the method, the diffusion slows down and the curve flattens *(Development of Medical Technology -Washington D.C -U.S. Government Printing Office. 1976)*. The diffusion may even drop due to demonstrated lack of benefit or the introduction of more effective technology e.g. the decline of the operation of Prefrontal leucotomy for obsessive compulsive neurosis, nephropaxy for floating kidney, ligating the internal mammary artery for angina, H2 receptor antagonists and proton pump inhibitors in great part replacing surgery in the treatment of peptic ulceration.

One should not expect this pattern to be universally applicable to the use of any new technology. The introduction of a new diagnostic or therapeutic method often traces a different pattern. The initial diffidence is followed by a surge of enthusiasm (so far this is akin to the sigmoid curve). However, the subsequent widespread use of the method, at times inappropriately due to the learning curve, and perhaps by not-so-qualified clinicians, leads to its falling out of favour. The recognition of the proper indications, limitations and contra indications of the therapeutic method will lead to a more balanced use of the method concerned. This pattern is not a contradiction of the sigmoid curve, which deals with the speed of diffusion of a technology. The latter pattern deals with the actual frequency of utilisation, or popularity, of the method. The adoption and utilisation of a new technology usually occurs in stages described as the Innovation-Decision System *(Rodgers and Shoemaker)*:

(i)   Awareness -   the potential adopter learns about the new therapeutic method

(ii) Trial - the adopter tries it out on a limited basis

(iii) Decision - the adopter decides to accept or reject it

(iv) Confirmation - the adopter seeks reinforcement for his decision, which may take the form of a 'blessing' by the authorities or peers.

Awareness of these patterns should induce the surgeon to be more scientific in his attitude to new therapies and technologies, rather than indulge in rigid and negative conservatism, or at the other extreme, uncritical enthusiasm. In practice one should seek to learn about new technologies, but these should be approached cautiously, discouraging their widespread use until reliable evidence of benefit becomes available. Universal agreement on the setting of priorities in the implementation of new technologies and fair sharing of medical resources is notoriously difficult. Devising principles for rationing that should govern the setting of priorities ahead of time has proved too general and difficult to apply in practice. A different approach, termed 'accountability for reasonableness', has been proposed by Norman Daniels. This involves transparency about the grounds for decisions, valid reasoning that is universally accepted, feasibility and clear pathways for appeals and revisions of decisions. This is done in real time as one faces the actual problems. One must note however, that 'grounds for decisions' and 'valid reasoning' involve premises, syllogisms and therefore principles. The difference between these two methods lies in generalisation and timing.

Learning curves of a new technique or technology involve (i) the individual surgeon, (ii) the institution where the new technique is introduced and (iii) the national and international specialist community. Tracker trials and clinical ethical committees, which take learning curves into consideration, can help in identifying treatments that perform poorly. Their aim is to minimise the risk to the individual patient who gives his informed consent for a new therapy, while maximising the potential for experience by the operator and the benefit to other similar patients. The institution where such procedures are carried out should have an acceptable record in the particular field and sufficient catchment to allow rapid learning. Thus, new techniques should be introduced in a limited number of centres, for a sufficiently long period of time, preferably having teams of surgeons of equivalent skill and experience working and learning in collaboration. Needless to say, the results should be carefully monitored *(Bull, C., Yates, R., Sarkar, D., Deanfield, J., de Leval, M.)*.

Broad Criteria for Adoption of New Technologies

These may be considered under three headings:

(a) Technical accuracy – The intrinsic value of the technology used.

(b) Clinical validity – The applicability of the technology to clinical practice e.g. ease of use, which includes reliability, rapidity of favourable action, accessibility, robustness, cost and, in the case of diagnostic technologies, ease of interpretation.

(c) Clinical utility – The potential for improving the clinical outcome when compared with existing therapies. This involves consideration of the sensitivity and selectivity of the technology, as well as the probabilistic nature of its effects.

Factors which Influence Adoption of New Technologies

Clinical factors: These include:

The severity of the disease being treated.

The availability of the new technology.

The availability and effects of alternative treatment.

The possibility of surveillance for the effect of the new technology.

The clinical consequences of the use of the new technology.

The clinical consequences of the adverse effects.

Social factors: These include: discovery, development, licensing, marketing factors, as well as economic, regulatory, ethical, legal and health service system considerations.

In order to maximise the utility of a technology, the clinician must possess some understanding of the physical, chemical or biological principles underlying the technology used in a given clinical situation. He must be aware of the advantages and disadvantages of the particular technological solution compared with alternatives, including cost considerations. Clinicians do not often consciously apply the principles of basic sciences. They apply (or should apply) these subconsciously, because these principles become ingrained in their thought processes. In fact, the greater the mastery of these principles, the less is the need for a conscious effort in their application. This emphasizes even further the necessity for clinicians to have a good grounding in the basic sciences. One must resist the temptation to adopt the latest technology because this fascinates the clinician or impresses the patient. Furthermore one must not deceive patients by using latest high-technology terms (e.g. laser) when in fact one is referring to more established but older technology (e.g. radio frequency), taking advantage of the patient's ingenuity.

The development of a new health technology calls for assessment as to when it can be regarded as an accepted routine procedure. Because of the variety and complexity of these innovative technologies, one cannot hope to develop one single formula for such an assessment. Even the timing of such an assessment may be controversial, in that, a technology can only be assessed when its users have gone beyond the learning curve for a particular technique and by then, assessments such as randomised trials may be considered unethical *(Mowatt, G., Bower, D., Brehner, J., Cavins, J.A., Grant, A., McKee, L.)*.
One practical solution to this problem would be continuous evaluation of technical innovations. The following algorithm illustrates the method:

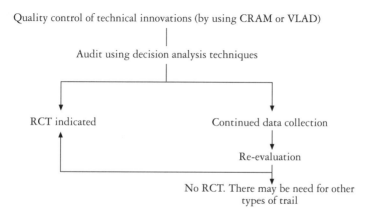

It is helpful to apply a few simple rules prior to the introduction of new developments:
(i)   Analysis of potential harms and benefits.
(ii) Independent close surveillance.
(iii) One must be very careful when dealing with disease prevention in healthy subjects, and with expressions of medicalization.
(iv) One must always keep in mind that lack of evidence of harm is not the same as evidence that no harm results.
Though these points would seem empirical, lessons from past and present, e.g. the relationship of HRT to breast cancer (The million women study collaborators) *(Mayor S)* and to the risk of myocardial infarction, are seemingly difficult to digest.

The Media and New Medical Technologies
The media tend to adopt different attitudes in respect to new technologies, at different times. They emphasise the positive aspects in its early stages and then highlight negative effects at a later stage, which are often illustrated as sensational

personal narratives. Examples of this abound: The side effects of the measles-mumps-rubella vaccine; the rise and fall of the contraceptive implant Norplant; the use of human albumin in shock and innumerable other cases. Overoptimistic reviews in the media could foster demand for inappropriate interventions and lead to iatrogenic harm, increased dissatisfaction, disillusionment or despair and unnecessary cost *(Coulter, A.)*. This is exemplified by the Di Bella debate in Italy and the 'mushroom-cure' incident on the local scene. The media are often carried away by the sensational results of research, which have not been corroborated by other properly conducted trials. One further example of this is the way autologous bone marrow transplantation for the treatment of breast cancer, was presented as a breakthrough, with major medical, social and legal consequences. In 1991, a California Court of Law ruled in favour of 89 million USD in damages, for having been refused this treatment on the basis of the results of one uncorroborated scientific publication but wildly enthusiastic reports in the lay press. By 1999 several major randomised trials failed to support the use of the above technique *(Lotz, J.P., Peters, W.)*. Media coverage of mass disasters offers another example where misinformation leads to mistakes in management: The insistence that cadavers constitute a major public health threat is often repeated but has no scientific basis. To direct a proportion of the human resources to tackle this problem as a priority is a mistake since it detracts from more urgent, effective and beneficial pursuits and may, in itself, create social problems, such as, lack of death certification and the inability of relatives to honour their dead. Proper resumption of public services, such as, attention to the safety of water and food, immunization, disposal of waste and sanitation, are surely more urgent and important *(de Ville de Goyet, C.)*. The right type of emphasis by the media would surely help. A strategy aimed at avoiding misinformation of the public requires investment in specialist training of information providers and materials.

Even where there is no active misinformation, the public may opt for unproven therapies through errors of logic, psychological, social and cultural reasons, as exemplified by some attitudes towards unproven aspects of alternative medicine. These include mysticism, belief in the superiority of 'natural' products, anti-scientific attitude, the will to believe, wishful thinking, the fallacy of the consequent, the illusion that a therapy works when other factors are at work e.g. the natural history of the disease, spontaneous remission, placebo effect and misdiagnosis *(Beyerstein, B.L.)*.

Improving Health Care
One can attempt to improve health care by: (i) Increasing resources (does health care merit a greater share of the GNP?) (ii) Increasing efficiency. (iii) Adopting the right priorities. Since no health system is 100% efficient, setting priorities is one tool aimed at optimising investment in health. Present policies of cost containment,

which will probably remain with us for some time, necessarily impose allocation of priorities. There are times when a conflict arises between financial constraints and long term economic sense, as well as, between these and individual and collective patients' rights. One can attempt to resolve these problems by using comparative analysis techniques of new versus old technologies, cost-benefit analysis comparing both cost and effectiveness as well as quality of life considerations, correcting the length of life to 'life of good quality' experienced by the patient. It has already been pointed out that the application of cost benefit analysis to surgery can be difficult and even of doubtful morality e.g. should one use expensive high technology on patients with poor prognosis and consequently expect a poor return. This point is so crucial in the discussion of priority-setting and the use of limited resources, that this emphasis through repetition is justified. It is easy for the private medical sector to refrain from providing such treatment as long as the public sector takes on the onus, but it is not easy to see how state medicine could, in all conscience, adopt similar attitudes. This will necessarily result in the shifting of the sicker, more expensive, prognostically worse patients to public institutions with obvious artificially adverse effect on their cost-benefit record. Everybody would agree that citizens are expected to respect the law of the land irrespective of their age, state of health, life expectancy etc. Then why should we use these same factors as discriminating points in health policy decisions? The limitations of certainty in medicine, the individual variation of patients and the need for judgement at an individual level, has led to a change of emphasis. The responsibility for priority-setting, has been shifted to grass roots i.e. district health authorities, clinicians and patients, away from central policy making. It is important to have constructive and transparent dialogue between the interested parts in an independent setting *(Kleinert, S.).*

Rehabilitation

Rehabilitation requires a multidisciplinary, problem- oriented approach, which goes beyond the domains of surgery and medicine, well into the social sphere. It is an often underestimated and forgotten aspect of therapy. Considering the fact that 13-14% of the population in western countries and probably more in third world countries, carry a degree of disability, this attitude is totally illogical and incomprehensible *(Badley, E.M., Tennant, A.).*

The emphasis lies on goal-setting and multiprofessional teamwork involving co-ordination, expertise and education. Admittedly, the medical or surgical condition will influence the outcome of rehabilitation, but the process has become the antithesis of medicalisation, going beyond a mechanistic extension of medicine into other, especially social, fields *(Wade, D.T., de Jong, B.A.).*

Self-reported Health

Measures of self-reported health e.g. simple global questions or more complex assessments of quality of life are considered important for assessment of outcomes of treatments and management strategies. In fact self-reported health (SRH) is also a good predictor of clinical outcome. Other application of SRH include screening for high-risk groups and as an endpoint for clinical trials. It is difficult to explain how an answer to a simple global question could be so useful and important. Perhaps, an early perception by the patient of early symptoms or signs of progression of their disease, which are not clinically evident or even generally considered of prognostic importance, may be one reason *(Fayers, P.M., Sprangers, M.A.G.)*.

The Health Care Pyramid

This is composed of the health of the population at the very base, going through self- care, primary health care, secondary health care, with tertiary health care at its apex. Relatively small changes towards the base result in significant demands at higher levels. Since only one in every forty symptoms ever reach medical consultation, *(Jones, R.)*, it is obvious that the quality of health care is of paramount importance for the significant proportion of people who at some time or other, deal with their own symptoms. Improvement in this level of care should not be in conflict with attempts to improve access to higher levels, especially when one considers cost–benefit and resource–availability aspects. Management of the interface between self-care and primary health care merits more consideration.

Manpower planning in the various strata of the health care pyramid is notoriously difficult and often results in projections, which are off the mark. One of the reasons for this is that one cannot rely entirely on complicated mathematical formulae for these projections since these do not take into account such important variables as low morale and disenchantment with the system, which may lead to poor and low volume outputs as well as resignations and collapse of any system.

Decision Making in Health Care

Policy makers in Health Services as well as clinicians are subjected to three types of pressures when making clinical and policy decisions:

(i)   Raising standards of care
(ii) Economic constraints i.e. careful use of health care resources, thus increasing efficiency.
(iii) Maintaining and improving equity.

The principal objective of a Health Service is to maximize the aggregate improvement in the health status of the whole community, that is, maximize the quality of life and the life expectancy. As a result the clinician often has to adapt more cost-effective forms of management, though this is often a cause of practical and moral concern. The percentage of public expenditure on pharmaceuticals in relation to the gross national product in countries belonging to OECD (Organisation for Economic Co-operation and Development) has risen from 0.4% in 1970 to 0.7% in1996, i.e. an increase of about 50%.this is great news for the shareholders of the major pharmaceutical companies, not so much for the providers and consumers of health care *(Freemantle, N., Hill, S.)*.

Even a genuine breakthrough in medical technology can create a dilemma for the clinician who has to decide whether the benefits thereof justify the usual increased costs of the procedures. A relocation of funds in the direction of the new technology might well result in decreased care for patients with other surgical problems. Distribution of resources cannot be solely based on principles of fairness e.g. a scarce resource can be distributed fairly by withholding it from one and all!

Cost–benefit Analysis

Cost-benefit analysis evaluates the cost of a course of action against the benefits likely to result from it in terms of cash savings, lives saved, years of life gained, working hours saved, health care support avoided, loss of earnings, care of dependants, compensation claims avoided, and much more difficult to assess, improvement in the quality of life *(Butt, W., Newhauson, D.)*. This is a method for plotting the points on a curve, quantifying the direction of change in quality and cost that occurs with alternative modes of diagnosis and treatment. It is not intended for the instances where cost increases and quality of care decreases, or where cost decreases and quality of care and results increase. These do not require analysis. Its real role is to assign a tangible value to instances where the cost as well as quality of care both increase i.e. in cases of unidirectional changes in quality and cost *(Rhodes, R.S., Rhodes, P.)*.

The economic costs and benefits of any aspect of medical management may be assessed by three methods: cost-benefit analysis (CBA), cost-effectiveness analysis (CEA), and cost-utility analysis (CUA). Cost-benefit analysis is the gold standard where all the costs and benefits of a procedure are listed and discounted to the year zero. Cost-effectiveness analysis expresses the net direct and indirect costs and cost savings in terms of a predefined unit of health outcome. Cost-utility analysis assesses health outcomes in terms of utility or quality, e.g. quality-adjusted life years (QALY) and disability-adjusted life years (DALY) *(Meltzer, M.I.)*.

Cost-efficacy is obviously only one factor in the equation of decision making in surgical or healthcare management. Health is the responsibility of society as a whole. The reduction in investment in state healthcare, in the name of cost-effectiveness, may well result in shunting of inadequately paid health workers and frightened patients to the private sectors. Though this may, (or perhaps may not), make cost-benefit sense in reducing the load on the state service, it is surely a moral and intellectual loss. A proportion of valid health-workers are driven into a system where self-interest prevails over the care for those who the private sector ignores.

Furthermore, quantifying the 'benefit' in cost-benefit analysis is a problem: The question 'which is the most beneficial treatment for the patient?' is not the same as 'which patient is it most beneficial to treat?' In other words, it is not easy to balance need and benefit.

A case has been made for the introduction of disease management programmes to improve health outcomes in a cost-efficacious manner in chronic high-cost diseases such as asthma and diabetes mellitus. This implies joint ventures and contracting out services between governments and industry as well doctors and industry. The possible hazards in this initiative include fragmentation of care with its undesirable sequelae, possible increase in cost after an initial period of cost-containment (drug company shareholders are not essentially philanthropists) and decreased professional independence of health workers contracted on a commercial basis. Besides the exercise could serve as a marketing ploy for the unscrupulous entrepreneur *(Richards T)*. The road to hell is paved with good intentions.

Inter–professional Cooperation

The awareness of the complexity of diseases and patients' needs has led to increased areas of interfaces between health professionals in different fields and indeed between health and other professionals having shared goals focused on patients' needs and leading to a more intense and altruistic team spirit in true inter-professional collaboration. This should overcome the obvious psychological, cultural and social barriers to such a team effort. A modification of undergraduate medical training in this direction would be necessary for this to become effective. Theoretically, one would expect an improvement in cost efficacy, though hard evidence for this is scanty *(Weiss, K.B., Mendosa, G., Schall, M.W., Berwick, D.B., Roessner, J.)*. Such collaboration requires good leadership. It takes a full orchestra to play a symphony, but it needs a good conductor to get it right.

Such teamwork will surely improve the knowledge the professionals have of one another's fields and methods, which can only have positive results. The learning of such techniques and strategies in collaboration between professionals cannot but help in improving one's abilities to communicate and collaborate with patients, which also involves a mutual understanding of the uncertain nature of surgical decision making and management.

It is important to realise that the clinical process is probabilistic and imprecise resulting in a certain degree of uncertainty. This uncertainty has different sources: One tries to remedy collective uncertainty through research, individual uncertainty through education, training and aids (see Chapter 2) and use communication to minimise the adverse effects of uncertainty resulting from chance. Statistical data should be honestly interpreted into useful information for discussion with patients, perhaps comparing the clinical situation and its risks to everyday life situations. One should avoid manipulating the patient towards one's pre-conceived ideas, though this is obviously difficult. One can use aids such as booklets, video-tapes, interactive computer programmes, accepting the fact that all this requires time. There is often a distinct difference between the outcome of treatment, the surgeon's perception of this and the patient's expectations. Satisfaction with a service depends on the relationship between expectations and reality. Transparency about availability, cost-effectiveness, options and results is obviously an important aspect of inducing realistic expectations. The problem is that there is a price to pay for all medical and surgical procedures and in that price is the source of dissatisfaction with the clinical process.

Prescribing Information

Patients have a right to be given factual, supportable, understandable and appropriate information, to allow them to decide whether they wish to receive therapy (WHO Assembly Decleration, 1994).

This implies that patients have a right to prescribing information of medicines and prescribers have a duty to explain. This is to an extent achieved through a printed information leaflet (PIL) and this is fast becoming the basis of the therapeutic dialogue between prescriber and patient. The prescriber's knowledge of the contents of PILs is being taken as a legal standard of competence *(Collier, J.)*. A computer program that delivers the latest relevant research regarding the commonest prescribed medications, at the actual moment of prescribing, including drug alerts, is now available *(Larkin, M.)*.

Thus PILs have to be up to date, readable and reliable, avoiding vague terminology. In this respect it is probably more effective to pinpoint common and serious side-effects, avoiding rarities and minutae, whilst giving an indication of the percentage risk involved.

Despite all the good intentions, errors in the use of medicines occur and are on the increase. The reasons for this include: an increased clinical load resulting in shorter consultation times, a steady stream of new drugs, super-specialisation resulting in a narrower knowledge base, the increased use of drug therapy over the years, an aging population a larger proportion of which is more sensitive to the adverse effects of drugs and the complexity of drug-drug interaction which is difficult to master even with sufficiency. It is obvious that no system can protect us from errors and mishaps of drug use, the source of which, may be the prescriber, the dispenser or the consumer of the medication.

Ethical Considerations and Patient Rights

There are recognised obligations of clinicians and medical practitioners in general, as well as patient rights, which where originally enshrined in tradition but which have now been formalised as international conventions.

The International code of Medical Ethics is based on the Hippocratic Oath (see

'Quotations' earlier on in this chapter), as updated in the Declaration of Geneva, 1947. This document was further amended by the 22nd and 35th World Medical Assembly in1968 and 1983 respectively. The WMA has considered and published material on a number of ethical matters which include: Discrimination in medicine, Rights of the patient, Human experimentation, Therapeutic abortion, Medical secrecy, Uses of computers in medicine, Torture and other cruel, inhuman and degrading treatments or punishment and Terminal illness.

The balance of professional obligations (beneficence) and patient rights (autonomy) is reflected in the doctor - patient relationship. Both these aspects are of the utmost importance in considerations on medical management, though there has been more emphasis on patient rights in recent years. Rights are related to justice and justice is founded on fairness and equity. The U.N. Committee on Economic, Social and Cultural Rights has started the process of devising guidelines for the design, implementation and monitoring of governmental and intergovernmental obligations regarding people's right to health, under the umbrella of human rights treaties. This process is still in the stage of 'general comment' *(Loff, B., Grustin, S.).*

Deciding on moral issues in medicine should not fall squarely on single categories, whether they are medical, legal or ecclesiastical, but rather, there should be a dialogue amongst all concerned in the issues, including the professions and the medical consumers *(Mallia, P.).*

Conclusion

We often hear commonplace remarks on surgical treatment the likes of 'The patient has a diseased organ – the surgeon chops it off.' In fact, most forms of treatment in surgical practice are merely aimed at giving nature half a chance to deal with the disease process. Such treatment is admittedly at a 'bow-and-arrow stage' as regards the technology employed, e.g. surgeons still use needle and 'thread' to suture tissues while the housewife has been using sewing machines for over one and a half centuries and industry has been using fast-acting glues for decades. Archaic though it may appear, treatment in surgical practice has to follow the pathways of logic, basing on present knowledge or theories of the mechanisms of disease. It is well to stress that though there is no hard and fast line distinguishing knowledge (fact) and theory, the latter are really works of the imagination which come into and fall out of fashion, maybe to become fashionable again years later. Surgical treatment is based on theories and tends to follow suit, not always to the patients' advantage. Patients may do well because of our treatment; sometimes in spite of it.

Chapter 5

Maintaining Competence

Quotations:
Hippocrates (ca 460-337 BC): 'The life so short, the craft so long to learn'.
Professor Edward Teller (Nuclear physicist, 1908 -): 'An expert is one who has made all possible errors in a small field'.

History

Influenced by the teachings of Socrates, Plato and Hippocrates, Aristotle helped to establish the Theory of Disease based on four humours; (i) blood, (ii) phlegm, (iii) white bile and (iv) black bile (leading to sanguine, phlegmatic, choleric and melancholic temperaments), four qualities i.e. hot, cold, moist and dry, and four types of matter i.e. earth, air, fire and water. It took our best medical brains, millennia to test, let alone contest, the validity of these 'undeniable axioms'. More recently there has been a reversal of the entrenched, centuries old belief that neurons in the adult human brain cannot undergo mitosis *(Gage, F.H. et al.)*. This is an eye-opener, a lesson to learn, in our endeavours to maintain competence.

The Dutch physician, teacher and chemist Boerhaave (1668-1738) proposed the following idea of scientific method 'When a medical problem presents itself, not accountable but upon hypothesis, we should restrain our judgement and leave the doubt to be solved by posterity, when they shall have obtained light enough from experiments which have escaped us. It therefore behoves us to defer our opinion about .... till time shall bring the truth to light. By this means Physic (Medicine) will be reduced to a small compass, but than it will be true, certain and always the same'. (U–205 Course Team. 1985. Boerhaave 1708, quoted in Medical Knowledge: Doubt & Certainty. Open University Press.).

We are thus encouraged to stick to certainty and to distinguish beliefs from knowledge - a sceptical attitude to science. The 'limit' proposed by Boerhaave where scientific (including medical) data were all certainties, may occur in an ideal world, but, alas, we have to base our judgement and decisions very often on probabilities and trade- offs or combinations of these using practical reasoning in contradistinction to theoretical reasoning (vide. Chap.1). We do need scientific knowledge but we also need what used to be vaguely called 'wisdom'. On the other hand Boerhaave's statement delivers the idea that to get at the truth we must test it, and that this is a slow, painstaking process of learning, which is however worthwhile. For the physician and the surgeon, this search must be lifelong, and the basic necessity of this is to be able to shamelessly admit the limitations of our 'certainties' One must admit that all research and clinical work involves subjective perception, and so different methods, and, perhaps, different operators, produce different perspectives. To make the effort worthwhile, one has to assume an underlying reality, which can be studied and a 'truth' which, though unreachable, the researcher tries his best to approach.

The idea of a body of trained professionals sharing collectively in the best scientific knowledge of their day and drawing their medical authority from membership of this group or college, took root in Italy in the late fifteenth century. Over the centuries more and more medical practitioners worldwide were embraced by the professional, scientific ethos and recognised as members by accredited bodies, the 'guardians of the colleges' which guarded access to the colleges, vetted what was to be considered as knowledge and expelled those considered guilty of unprofessional conduct. Modern medicine derives its authority in part from this monopoly of collective 'scientifically generated knowledge'. This process is relatively recent: The first recorded medical conference was held in Paris in1867.

Professional Development

Putting the idea of authority aside, we need this collective scientifically generated 'knowledge' to use as the basis of our practical reasoning in tackling the uncertainty of surgery *(Bursztajn, et al.)*. It is our duty to accumulate, critically evaluate, discard, store or use these data as they emerge to the best of our ability.

It is sometimes distressing to find different schools of medical thought proposing conflicting and even contradictory ideas and techniques. On the other hand, the establishment of international tertiary education centres, which originate and are controlled by one state or school of thought, as well as the adoption of standard information technology courses, carries an inherent danger. The centre with the best technological backup will eventually monopolise the rest, but it dose not necessarily follow that the best ideas emanate from such a centre. It is difficult to imagine how such a system could foster cross-fertilisation of ideas, which is so important for development and improvement in the medical field.

In our quest for professional development and improvement the three-stage model of Egan is applicable: One assesses the present situation, imagines the goal, then devises methods which allow passage from the first to the second consideration *(Egan, G.)*. Medical students, doctors and specialists are subjected to forces, which shape their continuing professional development. These include:

(a) The development of new medical data, hypothesis and techniques. These new developments are not neutral and may have bad as well as good effects, increasing suffering rather then reducing it e.g. the Thalidomide disaster. These new data may not be limited to developments in the medical field. Medical and surgical practice is also affected by developments in other fields e.g. modern physics and mathematics, in the same way that any field of science may benefit from advances in other branches. Powerful quantum computers which are not restricted by the 0 and 1 binary code intrinsic to silicon chip computers are in the phase of development as a result of physics research on the slowing of the speed of light to zero *(Mitton, S.)*. One can imagine how these developments can affect the evolution of medical technology.

(b) The evolution of 'evidence' and the consequent reaction of the medical profession e.g. the data regarding the merits and demerits of HRT, reflect the inherent difficulties and flaws in our methods of producing, disseminating and assimilating evidence. There are various reasons for this:

(i) Interpretation of evidence is subjective to a degree.

(ii) Critical evaluation is sometimes scientifically lacking.

(iii) Entrenched beliefs are not easily discarded in favour of new evidence.

(iv) Clinicians dealing with a restricted number of patients may have difficulty in having the same perspectives as scientists dealing with vast statistics.

(v) The pharmaceutical and medical technology industries, faced with negative research, may seek to control the damage by raising doubts and creating confusion.

(vi) The media thrive on the sensational and enthusiastic reports at one time may turn into alarmist reporting later.

(vii) The negative potential of the influence of industry on published research, as well as conflicts of interest of researchers.

(viii) Ignored biases and confounding.

(c) Changes in the character and incidence of disease e.g. Scarlet fever was a severe and commonly lethal disease decades ago, but became mild even before the advent of antibiotics. Diabetes used to be a chronic disease of relatively short duration since the victims did not live long. After the introduction of insulin it most commonly manifests itself in its long-term complications or in the iatrogenic manifestation of hypoglycaemia. Rheumatic fever is another disease, which has changed within our professional lifetime. A further example is the development of antibiotic resistance by micro-organisms and the various methods of genetic transfer of this resistance (refer to Chapter 4: Antibiotics in the treatment of surgical infection), which is a source of concern and a stimulus to find strategies which prevent us from being out-smarted by microbes.

(d) Changes in human society leading to new disease, new methods of transmission etc. Examples are the transmission of tropical diseases to unexpected locations, AIDS, radiation effects of the Chernobyl disaster, effects of civil and military strife.

(e) Medicalisation – medical jurisdiction has expanded and now encompasses many problems e.g. alcoholism, homosexuality etc. which did not previously fall within its sphere of influence *(Williams, S.J., Colnan, M.)*.

The Influence of Other Disciplines

Apart from the factors to which we have just referred, there are also problems arising out of the intrinsically complex nature of disease and our concept of this in the light of tradition: The sharp division between what is somatic (natural science based) and what is psychological has its roots in the traditional Cartesian division of 'res cogitans' (thinking substance) and 'res extensa' (corporeal substance). In fact, the human body is not simply composed of organs, cells and electron microscopic cellular organelles, but may be thought of as molecules, atoms and eventually sub atomic structures or elementary particles. The latter can be considered akin to Plato's 'forms' *(Heisenberg, W.)* or even as mathematical structures. This may be considered as an expression of 'reductionism', which is the process whereby a relatively autonomous theory becomes absorbed by, or reduced to, some other more inclusive theory, when the laws of the secondary theory or science are shown to be logical sequences of the primary science *(Velanovich, V.)*. Thus, considering a hierarchy in biological sciences one could consider the following order: (i) Mathematical structures (ii) Elementary particles (iii) Atoms (iv) Molecules (v) Electron-microscopic cellular organelles (vi) Cells (vii) Organs (viii) Individuals (ix) Populations (x) Races (xi) Species. Autonomous sciences develop at each of these levels, e.g. molecular biology and biochemistry correspond to the molecular level; histology at organ level. However, some sciences, including medicine, involve more than one level. Despite this, the application of reductionism to medicine is still a logical possibility. The probabilistic nature of the clinical process results, amongst other things, from the fact that patients are 'wholes', which are to a degree distinct and different and this renders the application of reductionism to medicine, at least, difficult.

It is appropriate to point out at this stage, risking a slight digression, that though Rene' Descartes certainly did stress the distinction between the mind and the body in his 'Meditations on First Philosophy' *(Veitch, J.)*, more specifically in his Second and Sixth Meditation, he was equally clearly aware of the unity and interdependence of the psychological and the somatic. This comes out clearly in the Sixth Meditation. Body function is an expression of the mind, just as the mind is an expression of the body. Thus, the strict division between 'res cogitans' and 'res extensa' and consequently between 'psyche and 'soma' does not hold. This had been underlined by Thomas Aquinas and is evidenced by a multitude of psychosomatic diseases e.g. aerophagy, irritable bowel syndrome, etc. Research evidence also supports this view and has been already discussed in more detail under 'Management of Functional Somatic Symptoms' in Chapter 4. *(Kamolz, T., Bammer, T., Pointner, R.), (Felice, A.).* The brain or mind may alter the way pain-producing information is processed, effecting not only perception but also body response. In this respect one needs to elaborate on the traditional division between brain and mind, which is deeply rooted in the nineteenth century division between neurology and psychiatry. This is again

To do: 1) order 'through the looking Glass' for Amber
2) Organise wheels for ½ turn (Benny?)
3) Uma cançõo pure Lole.

Maintaining Competence 157

a misleading division. The pathological processes involved are interdependent and both are potentially influenced by social and environmental factors. The close connection between brain and mind is not reflected in the attitudes of neurologists and psychiatrists.

Medicine must adapt to developments in modern physics, other basic sciences and philosophy, which form its natural scientific base *(Schmahl, F.W., von Weizsacher, C.F.)*. Advances in other fields of knowledge may also produce a more than tangential effect on attitudes in the medical field.

Academia and Clinical Skills

Because of the importance given to experience in research when surgeons apply for jobs or promotions, it is customary for surgeons in training to take a two or three year break to pursue pure clinical research. Taking time-off to indulge in pure or clinical research can result in loss of clinical skills, especially in skill-intensive specialities such as surgery. This is more marked if the time for acquiring skills before this deviation into research is relatively short *(Taylor, I.)*. One could enjoy the best of both worlds if part-time clinical, part-time research assignments were organised, perhaps over a longer time period. These clinician-scientist posts should enable research oriented clinical academics to further their clinical training while helping them to secure key academic posts. This will help encourage recruitment and retention of expertise even on the academic side. Though one should reward excellence in teaching, which is essential for the production of better doctors, setting up a timetable of intensive teaching for doctors involved in research, will surely affect the latter activity adversely. Perhaps too much emphasis is being placed on research-potential at the expense of clinical and teaching abilities when jobs are allocated. If a more appropriate balance is struck in the evaluation of all these useful potentials, this will influence the surgical market forces to the advantage of the patient needing health care. If the academic surgeon is going to teach future practicing doctors, then his clinical and technical skills should be as important as they are to the Health Service surgeon. One could compromise by having three groups of medical academics:

(i) The research group.

(ii) The clinician-educator group, involved with formal and clinical teaching.

(iii) The associated clinical group, primarily involved with clinical practice but also help with clinical teaching.

These three groups should not only interact, but there could be planned rotations between groups.

Medical Education

It is self evident that improvement in medical care requires adequate medical education. The hallmarks of medical education in the past were factual knowledge, regular exams, organised hands-on experience and apprenticeship. This was not a bad system, which however is suffering under the strain of a progressively expanding curriculum. Doctors are learners and teachers throughout their professional life. However most of us ignore medical educational research, which is mainly published in specialised journals. This is a self-inflicted handicap, which we must shake off if we seriously intend to tackle present and future challenges. One must keep in mind that different learning methods tend to suit different individuals and different learning needs. The teaching method should foster the student's ability to function and learn independently. This implies sensitivity on the part of the teacher to the student's need for guidance.

A medical curriculum may be considered at different levels: what is planned, what is delivered, what is experienced by the students, what is absorbed and what is applied. The gap between theory and practice can be bridged by adopting better and more practical teaching and learning methods, including basic forms of 'knowledge' e.g. thought processes and problem solving techniques, concentrating on enduring outcomes. The needs of the health service and of the community must be taken into consideration when planning curricula.

Integrated problem based curricula have been introduced in many centres. This involves the use of problem cases or situations leading to specific learning objectives, increasing knowledge and understanding as well as improving generic skills and method.. Though participants in this form of teaching may obtain more satisfaction than with traditional methods, there is no evidence that the output in knowledge, performance and patient outcomes is better *(Smits, P.B.A. et al.).* There is no advantage in terms of scores on standard exams or overall performance. In a study on the impact of student-generated learning carried out at the University of Maastricht, it was concluded that students exposed to problem-based curricula, seem to make better self-directed learners during their later years of training *(van den Hurk, M.M. et al.) (Norman, G.R., Schmidt, H.G.).* Careful analysis of the study, however, shows that this conclusion is not fully justified. It is possible to draw different interpretations and conclusions from the same data. There is also evidence that these students develop better cognitive abilities, self expression and even practical abilities at history taking and physical examination, *(Norman, G.R.), (Hmelo, C.E.),* resulting in better results in the clinical part of the examination and more propensity towards family medicine. This does not necessarily mean an improvement in the final product. This may be explained by the fact that expert knowledge is more extensive and better integrated than the content of problem based learning. It is a personal impression (unsupported by hard evidence) that students enjoy problem based learning more than traditional methods and find it easier to retain the material they learn. The teaching staff is, in general more favourable to problem based learning *(Albanese, M.A., Mitchell, S.).* On the other hand problem based curricula are relatively more expensive and it is doubtful whether this is justified by the resulting educational benefits.

Clinical tutorials are amongst the most effective methods of undergraduate teaching, presenting and discussing disease, or some of its aspects, in the context of a real patient and linking this to a discussion of the related theory and clinical reasoning. The fact that this method carries cognitive advantages has been experienced by countless generations of medical students and their teachers. This notion has considerable support in the relevant literature *(Burrows, H.S.)*. A recently proposed variation on the theme has been reported under the name of 'Clinical Reasoning Theatre' *(Borleffs, J.C.C. et al.)*, where the actors in the theatre are the patient, the doctor/teacher and the audience of students. The only relative innovation in this is perhaps the emphasis on the interaction between the three 'actors' in demonstrating clinical reasoning at the various stages of the clinical encounter. Even so, this feature was not foreign to the traditional clinical tutorials. This form of teaching is most fruitful if three conditions are satisfied: (i) Students must be assigned to clinical sites that foster the necessary learning experience. This is sometimes logistically difficult and needs careful planning. (ii) Teachers must take full advantage of the unique educational experiences provided by interactions with real patients in a clinical environment. (iii) One must ensure that the content of the teaching is clinically relevant.

There should be more emphasis on active learning and acquisition of clinical competence, which includes training in clinical thought and decision making, rather than passive acquisition and retention of facts. Educational programmes have to become more flexible with the learning of skills and assimilation of attitudes complimenting a core of knowledge. Student feedback and patient participation are essential. A higher degree intercalated at some stage in the medical course has the double advantage of encouraging academic and research potential and may serve as an acceptable escape track in case of a dropout later on in the course.

Most medical students and newly qualified doctors encounter difficulties when faced with the problem of career-selection. Self-selection remains stable with time in only about 20% of students *(Murdoch, M., Kressin, N., Fontier, L., Giuffre, P.A., Oswald, L.)*. Competent advice based on proper assessment and soun statistics would help the health service as well as the young doctors. The clinical and research activities of the clinical tutors should not restrict teaching activities and student contact if the medical school is to be a school. To be in a position to give reasonably adequate advice and direction in this respect, one must possess some measure of the students' values. These may include their bio-social orientation e.g. tendency towards consultative or longitudinal management, bio-scientific orientation e.g. technical or non-technical, academic interest, attitude towards prestige and income, attitude towards role strain, value placed on role support and manual dexterity including clumsiness factor *(Pulè, C.)*.

Methods of Assessment of Clinical Competence.

Competence, in the above context, is the ability to provide professional services in accordance with practice standards established by members of the profession and conforming to the expectations of society. This involves medical expertise, clinical decision making, communication skills, inter professional skills, collegiality, professionalism, willingness and ability to improve. This can hardly be determined than by critical observation of the student or clinician caring for patients in different clinical and environmental circumstances. Though an important part of any assessment of clinical competence should thus be based on these observations, which have been appropriately formalized and documented, this is not a robust way of assessing a doctor's clinical competence. The reason is that, unless strictly formalised, standards tend to be idiosyncratic since the definition of 'professional behaviour' is not widely shared and assessments are usually based on limited impressions on one or two dimensions. Furthermore there is a tendency to stress positive aspects rather than negative ones, leading to overgenerous evaluations. An objective structured exam, with all its disadvantages, is a helpful supplement to the workplace assessment.

Society, mostly through governmental bodies, assesses clinical competence by measuring healthcare processes and outcomes, as well as compliance with standards, guidelines and clinical service frameworks. These methods have evolved recently, most of the innovation coming from Canada *(Violato, C., Lockyer, J., Fidler, H.).* A multisource feedback system, in the form of a questionnaire, has been applied to the assessment of surgical competencies following its application to primary care clinicians and physicians.

Students tend to study the parts of the curriculum, which are assessable. Tests should therefore be tailor-made so that their content is conducive to learning objectives (blueprinting). With proper feedback tests would thus become educational and formative. In the written part of the assessment, different types of tests and formats are available each of which has its strong points and weaknesses:

The question's format is, however, of limited importance compared with its content in determining what the question tests. It is thus preferable if many different types of tests and formats are employed in order to assess such a multifactorial attribute as is clinical competence. Clear standards need to be defined, rather than relative norm referencing, adopting a minimum acceptable standard for each particular test.

The reliability of a test is a measure of its reproducibility and consistency. There are two aspects to test reliability: (i) Inter-rater reliability refers to consistency of rating by different examiners. This can be improved utilizing a larger number of examiners. (ii) Inter-case reliability i.e. variation from task to task. This is improved by broad sampling across cases. The validity of a test refers to the extent it succeeds in assessing the competencies for which it is designed.

Question Format	Advantages	Disadvantages
1) True or false questions.	Concise.	Difficult to construct absolutely true or false statements.
2) Single best option MCQ's.	Reliable i.e. accurate scoring. Easier to construct than true or false questions. Can test more than simple facts.	Not good for testing creativity, writing skills and hypothesising.
3) Multiple true or false questions (i.e. more than one correct answer).	Quite reliable.	Difficult to construct. Scoring is rather complicated.
4) Short answer open ended questions.	More flexible. Can test creativity and hypothesising. Useful for testing aspects of competence which cannot be otherwise tested.	Not good to assess factual knowledge. (Cannot cover a wide range of knowledge because they are time consuming to answer).
5) Essay questions.	Good for testing presentation, writing ability, reasoning and summarising.	Time consuming and so cannot test a wide range of knowledge. Limited reliability. (Difficult to score).
6) Key feature questions i.e. description of a realistic case followed by a number of questions that require straightforward answers.	Good for measuring problem solving abilities and application of knowledge. Good reliability and validity (i.e. it tests what it is supposed to test).	Time consuming to construct.
7) Extended matching questions. (This is composed of a list of options, and a lead-in question regarding one or more clinical situations, linked with the options.	Tests application of knowledge and problem solving more than MCQ's. Easy to score. Easier to construct than key feature questions. Good reliability.	Difficult to apply to certain themes. Time-consuming to answer when compared to MCQ's.

Figure: 5.1

In 1990 Miller conceptualised a pyramid of clinical competence. At the base of this pyramid there is knowledge of basic facts (Knows). At a higher level there is applied knowledge (Knows how). The third level refers to abilities in an experimental 'in-vitro' environment (Shows how), while the apex of the pyramid is the actual doctor's performance 'in-vivo' (Does).

The several types of assessments have their strong and weak points: MCQ's have a high reliability because of there wide application, but the knowledge tested may be trivial and does not stimulate active generation of knowledge. Essays and orals suffer from difficulty of consistent marking. All the above types of tests may be used to assess problem solving and clinical reasoning. Inter-case reliability can be improved by written formats having a large number of cases. In the viva-voce version, application is more difficult and unreliable. Computer simulations can replace written and verbal scenarios. The traditional clinical exam usually consists of one long case and a number of short cases. The problem here is that such tests cannot be standardised and if the examinee is not observed, one will be testing 'knows how' rather than 'shows how'. To achieve reliability the assessment must be sufficiently long and the number of cases should be large (as much as ten). One solution is the introduction of Observed Structured Long Examination Record (OSLER), where the candidate is observed interacting with the patient. Direct observation and sufficient test length are essential for validity. An alternative is Objective Structured Clinical Examination (OSCE). Here candidates rotate through a series of stations based on clinical skills applied to a range of contents. This provides multiple samples of performance, which can be assessed in addition to knowledge. This method is expensive and labour intensive. Besides, validity is limited by the short station length intrinsic to the method. Communication skills can be assessed using OSCE, but a great number of cases would be necessary (as many as 37) for validity (*Colliver, J.A. et al.*). Alternatively this can be assessed using patient assessment, but one wonders how consistent patients can be in such situations. Whether one uses global rating, scoring against checklists or patient-findings questionnaire (the latter mainly tests data-collecting abilities), trained examiners are essential to ensure consistency. The use of standardised patients, or even actors, requires extensive patient training and is consequently expensive. One can hardly imagine that it mirrors the conditions in real life. The assessment of in-vivo performance at the apex of Miller's pyramid is a problem, which has not been satisfactorily resolved. Continuous assessment and student portfolios attempt to measure the 'does' but there has been little research on the reliability and validity of these methods, not to mention their predictive value regarding subsequent clinical competence and educational role (*Wass, V., Van der Vleuten, Shatzer, N., Jones*).

Selection of Students for Medical School

This may be based on merit or on policy decisions promoting planned bias in favour of a particular social, ethnic or geographical group, to compensate for inequalities, or to cater more harmoniously for particular social groups in the catchment's population. It is obvious that these two criteria can easily come into conflict.

Interviews may help in assessing extra-academic merits, e.g. teamwork, leadership and social involvement. This is a positive thing were it not for the fact that it creates a bias towards those who had the opportunity to develop these qualities (*Tutton, P.*). A policy decision dictating quotas for a particular population group would predictably result in a high dropout rate in the quota group. The answer to the problem lies in the studied and planned reversal of whatever factors alienated the particular socio-economic, ethnic or geographical group. This having been achieved, the discussion of selection could then concentrate on the relative relevance of the many aspects of individual merit.

Clinical Evidence

There are several steps that intervene between the generation of new clinical evidence from research and its application into clinical practice. The new data is synthesised, leading to development of clinical policies or protocols (e.g. antibiotic policy), which then have to be applied clinically in the particular set-up. Evidence based practice aims at bridging the barriers between research evidence and clinical decision-making. Critical appraisal of evidence is based on the assessment of three main factors:

1. Validity – closeness to truth.
2. Importance – what effect will this new knowledge have?
3. Usefulness – how applicable is it to one's clinical situation?

The complaint of overload of students, teachers and practicing clinicians has been with us for decades and can only be solved by proper selection. IT smart searches could direct the practitioner once his pattern of practice has been established. One would however expect that this would eventually increase rather than decrease the doctor's load of relevant material. It is therefore essential to develop good judgement. There have been attempts at publishing critical appraisals of research, which have been already digested by 'experts' and are ready to be absorbed and applied by the busy clinician, e.g. The Cockrane Library (Haynes B and Haines A), 'Clinical Evidence' distributed by the NHS in UK and the United Health Foundation in the USA. Scientifically strong studies may be efficiently selected using Special Medline at a special screen, U.S. National Library of Medicine Clinical Queries, Ovid Technology Medline and Skolar Services. Journals of secondary publication e.g. Evidence Based Medicine and ACP Journal Club, serve this same purpose. They screen publications, publish structured abstracts, which are commented by authorities in the specific field. This may look efficient on the surface but carries the inherent danger of not giving enough information to the practising clinician to assess the value of the evidence of the research and the source. Thus, though quick access to accurate summaries of 'the best evidence' is improving, the clinician must guard against being reduced to a mindless pair of hands that automatically apply whatever the 'supreme experts' dish out, in an uncritical manner. Though the availability of these digests and clinical reviews reduces the need for going to the original articles, it does not, in effect, eliminate the difficulty to keep up with these syntheses *(Gyatt, G. et al.)*. This can hardly be considered as an advance in clinical practice in that there is a definite danger of abdication of responsibility by the intellectually lazy. Summaries and digests may help as an initial step, but research evidence that leads to alteration of established methods should lead the clinician to search deeper into the sources of the evidence and critically assess for himself what is 'best'. There are indications, that though printed handouts are certainly well intentioned and perhaps a step in the right direction, they are probably insufficient to alter doctors' practice significantly.

Though access has generally improved for some sections of the world scientific community, this does not apply for the poorer developing countries. The price of access has increased well beyond inflation and the value of information tends to increase as more people have access. Academics are trying to cooperate to make access more affordable *(Smith, R.)*. This together with the fact that some research can hardly be published in the usual printed article form, has encouraged the introduction of electronic publishing. This is a very cheap method of publishing and publishers will have to increase access to maintain profits. Electronic publishing initiatives such as Bio Med Central and Pub Med Central have strengths and weaknesses linked to their characteristic of minimal refereeing.

The most important factor in all this is the transferring of expert judgment to the recipient, a process which requires human interaction in addition to new technology, the availability of data and knowledge.

Evidence does not necessarily lead to innovation. Other synergistic initiatives are necessary to reach this desired goal of improved adoption of evidence. This includes educational outreach visits by opinion leaders, discussion with experts, academic detailing, targeted audit with feedback, computerised alerts and reminders and education in the adoption of evidence-based policies *(Barton, S.)*. Furthermore, even the best evidence requires sensible adaptation to the particular clinical situation.

The reduction in in-service training hours has complicated the issue of surgical training and competence even further and it is pertinent to investigate the most efficient methods of learning in surgery. Hands-on experience and problem solving seem to be the most popular with the trainees themselves *(Drew, P.J. et al.)*. These methods involve a time factor, which cannot be compressed beyond a certain limit. Reduction in working hours, though understandable, necessarily leads to longer periods of training. Improved efficiency of training content and method cannot completely eliminate this necessity. Reducing the breadth of surgical training in response to reduced training hours is clearly illogical and the results of such a decision would be unthinkable.

Best Practice
Any honest clinician will admit that all too often there are departures from what one considers as best practice:

(i) Health technologies which are yet unproven as to efficacy and safety are sometimes hastily adopted into everyday clinical practice e.g. rotoblader technique for recanalizing arteriosclerotic coronary arteries.

(ii) Methods and technologies, which are of proven effectiveness are too slowly introduced into clinical practice. A historical example was the delay in the acceptance of Lister's theory and technique of operative antisepsis.

(iii) A busy clinician does not have the time to evaluate each and every new technique or technology. Some statistical considerations mentioned earlier in this work spring to mind i.e.:

(a)   The knowledge base for a clinician is estimated to be over fifteen million facts and increasing daily.

(b)   The number of facts one can learn and retain is about nine facts per hour.

(c)   One can only remember and evaluate about seven concepts at any one time when confronted with a problem. (de Dombal)

(d)   To keep abreast of current advances one should read about 19 to 20 articles a day.

(e)   About 10,000 new RCT's are included in MEDLINE every year.

(f)   About 350,000 trials have been identified by the Cochrane collaboration.

(iv) The concept of 'best evidence' based on statistical considerations is more applicable to certain specialities and less to others e.g. the numerical component in a surgical study can hardly ever equal that in medicine and in public health: nor can surgical techniques be assessed in the same manner as medical therapy. A pill can be more efficiently standardised and crossed-over with a placebo than is possible in the case of surgical procedures!

(v)   Guidelines are often inadequate or indigestible.

Guidelines

Guidelines are useful in simplifying traditionally thorny problems. One example of a useful guideline of this type follows. This indicates clearly which investigative path to follow in different degrees of head injury:

1. Patients with normal conscious level, no signs of external injury and a history of trivial trauma, may be discharged home.

2. Patients who have lost consciousness, fallen over 60 cms. in height and who have a full thickness scalp laceration or other features of significant head trauma, loss of memory or are unable to give an adequate history, require a skull X-Ray.

3. In patients with a skull fracture a CT head scan is indicated.

Since the value of guidelines and recommendations is only as good as the judgments on which they are based, grading of the evidence and its interpretation is imperative. Explicit systematic attempts at grading the value of the evidence implied in guidelines have been attempted with some success (GRADE - Norway) in an honest effort to assess balance between benefits and harm, quality of evidence, applicability and risks.

There is an obvious need for bodies or institutions, which assess new and exciting health technologies, develop clear clinical guidelines and priorities, transmit them adequately to the health workers concerned and promote relevant and fair audit and clinical enquiries. Government and Health Institutions have a direct interest in promoting such bodies e.g. The National Institute for Clinical Excellence (NICE) in U.K. These bodies provide the Health Service with advice on the use of selected new and established technologies. Guidelines from such institutions are based on; (i) The clinical needs of patients in relation to other available technologies. (ii) Health Service priorities (a relative criterion). (iii) Cost-benefit considerations and relative effectiveness. (iv) Potential impact on other Health Service Resources. (v) The encouragement of innovation. (vi) Political decisions *(Rawlins, M.)*. To merit recommendation, the technology must be effective and good value for money. The best possible advice based on available data is given, with reservations about possible revision if and when new data becomes available. The criteria for such recommendations should be thoroughly discussed with clinicians. This will encourage acceptance and implementation provided the recommendations are practical and easily applicable. Transparent economic evaluation and studies of effectiveness cannot be left to the drug companies and should fall in the sphere of competence of bodies such as NICE. The problem arises when technologies are deemed effective but are particularly expensive, sometimes prohibitively so. Guidelines are also helpful when they expose technologies or techniques, which are not cost-effective, because resources can then be released for use for more effective pursuits. One has to accept that collecting and evaluating the data, which results in guidelines, costs money. This is money well spent if health workers make good use of valid advice.

There is better compliance in case of guidelines for acute care, when the quality of evidence is better, when the recommendations fall in line with existing values, when they are less complex, when the desired performance is clearly indicated and when they do not involve many new skills and organisational change.

There is good evidence that the use of clinical guidelines can change the process of health care and improve clinical outcomes *(Woolf, S.H. et al.)*. One example is the significant reduction in early complications of burns following compliance with guidelines in twenty U.S. emergency rooms *(Grimshaw, J.M., Russel, I.T.)*. These are not intended to cut costs or institute a form of rationing. For example an antibiotic policy will probably increase the costs in the short term by suggesting the introduction of newer more expensive antibiotics but may have cost containment effect long term by limiting misuse and encouraging the appropriate use of prophylactic rather than therapeutic methods. The intention is to encourage best practice and get good value for money. Even this laudable target may pose difficulties: The most honest and scientific of appraisals carries an element of judgement and therefore potential disagreement. Furthermore these assessments are based on data available at the time and further evidence may later emerge which contradicts the data, or the conclusions previously reached.

The volume of literature involving guidelines should be within the limits that clinicians can handle *(Tonks, A.)*. Guidelines must carry the potential to improve distinctly the quality of health care. They must themselves be subject to scrutiny of evidence and assessment of results and therefore have to be periodically and systematically revised. Updating of guidelines may be prompted by different situations: new information about the advantages or disadvantages of a technique or technology may become available; outcomes previously ignored, e.g. quality of life, become relevant; new diagnostic or therapeutic methods become available; when current practice is already near optimal; when there are changes in available resources *(Shekelle, P. et al.)*. The development, monitoring and appraisal of clinical guidelines needs a multidisciplinary basis and must differentiate between what is based on strong or on weak evidence. Feedback from clinicians is essential. The user should have enough information to assess the validity and applicability of the guideline *(Miller, J., Petrie, J.)*. Finally, the authors of guidelines should be free of competing interests or at least, declare them.

In this respect, a group of guideline authors, members of the Conference on Guideline Standardization (COGS), have published an 18-point check list for reporting clinical practice guidelines. These include description of targeted population, funding sources, pre-release review of information, potential benefits and harms, and barrier to the application of the recommendations. If kept simple these guidelines on guidelines should prove useful.

Factors which Influence the Uptake of Evidence
There are three basic considerations:
(i) The specific characteristics of the evidence i.e. its ease of adoption.
(ii) Barriers and facilitators of the process which can occur at various levels i.e. the patient, the clinician, the team, the organisation or at the level of society.
(iii) The effectiveness of the dissemination and implementation strategies.

Learning
Learning is a process, not an event. Adult learning follows a cyclical pattern illustrated below: Before one is aware of the changes in knowledge or technology, one is unconsciously incompetent and becomes consciously incompetent when he becomes aware of these. (Plate 6) Learning occurs when there is an attempt to exercise activities in new areas and with time and practice, becomes consciously competent. With even more practice, mastery develops and the individual becomes unconsciously competent or expert *(Leinster, S.J.)*.

Important to recognise

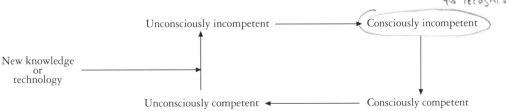

Plate 6

...from unconsciously incompetent

...to consciously incompetent

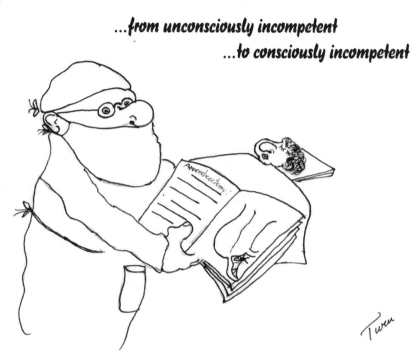

Clinicians generally learn by identifying the problem or need, finding the relevant resources, acquiring knowledge and gaining experience through practice and feedback *(Slotnick, H.B.)*.

Several models of learning styles have been proposed. The Kolb model describes four approaches to learning:

(a) Learning from concrete experience.

(b) Abstract conceptualisation with development of hypothesis, theories and analytical strategies.

(c) Active experimentation through action and risk-taking.

(d) Reflective observation i.e. seeing problems from multiple points of view resulting in a logical strategy of action.

The Tripartite model describes three approaches, as the name itself suggests:

(a) Deep learning, motivated by vocational interest, motivation and a search for deeper understanding and basic principles.

(b) Strategic learning, motivated by a desire to be successful and leading to patchy understanding.

(c) Surface learning motivated by fear of failure.

The learners could be categorised into four groups: The convergers who preferably use deductive methods, the assimilators who tend to use inductive methods of reasoning, the divergers who use creative problem-solving and the accommodators whose preferred method is hands-on experience.

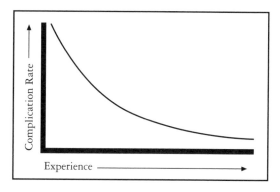

A learning curve is a graphic representation of the relationship between experience with a procedure and an outcome variable e.g. operative time, complication rate, hospital stay or mortality. The learning (performance) curve in surgery is steep in its early part and as experience accumulates, it becomes flatter, with less improvement with each additional experience. The shape of the learning curve is, as would be expected, different according to the learner and the task.

Quoting Bismarck, people (in our case clinicians) are hardly ever in full control of events; occasionally they are in a position to deflect them to their advantage. This is more likely to happen if one has an updated knowledge of these 'events'.

Medical students, doctors and specialists begin their clinical training and practice with a common knowledge base and basically a similar range of skills. In time this knowledge and these skills will vary appreciably. The knowledge of a physician tends to decline as a function of time as from graduation. This results more from failure to acquire new knowledge than from forgetting previously learnt material *(Day, S.C. et al.)*.

The continuous development of new data, hypothesis and techniques make the maintenance of competence in medicine in general, and perhaps more so in surgery, a moving target. This state of flux poses difficulties in an already probabilistic (not quite sure) atmosphere, but is also challenging and fascinating for the dedicated clinician. (There are clinicians who would prefer static and secure knowledge and practice, which does not change from the year tot - an obvious delusion). In our preoccupation with innovation we should not loose sight of ideas and techniques, which have proved their worth and stood the test of time. Continuing learning must be seen as a routine part of daily practice, which would be expected to lead to improved results. The most commonly encountered resistance to CME and CPD results from professional conservatism towards new learning methods *(Bashook, P.G., Parboosingh, J.)*. Objective evidence of quality of care can be obtained by integrating audit and self-assessment (including more frequent post-mortem examinations) into one's practice. Feedback on these results should not be seen as a threat but as an opportunity to learn. Even if results of such assessments are negative, they should point to remedial actions such as more intensive focused education or help from peers before resorting to punitive actions, such as suspending certification. The collection and analysis of performance data goes beyond the application of a few numerical tests of significance. A formal statistical quality control scheme e.g. the CRAM chart *(Poloniecki, Valencia, Littlejohns)* may give an early warning of adverse trends that may be followed up by more authoritative and in-depth investigations. Accurate and complete information regarding every stage of the clinical process (including costs and decision making at management level) is essential for clinical governance and continuous quality improvement. However, investment in information systems which are meant to collect, elaborate and diffuse this information, will only pay back if there is dedicated staff who will report this data promptly and accurately, as well as equally motivated doctors who will transfer this data into tangible results.

The Gaussian (Normal o Bell-Shaped) Curve

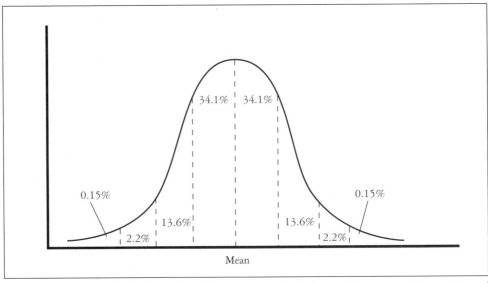

This is smooth, bell-shaped and is symmetrical about the mean. The point of inflection is that point where the curve changes from convex to concave. The standard deviation is the horizontal distance from the mean and the point of inflection on the curve.

Surgical Expertise
Determinants of surgical performance include technical skill, thorough training, compassion, sound judgement, communication skills, clinical acumen, knowledge, the collaborating team and good leadership. One must admit that one cannot expect to have surgeons who perform equally well or badly. Surgical expertise and performance can be expressed as a Gaussian curve with some surgeons having the best results.

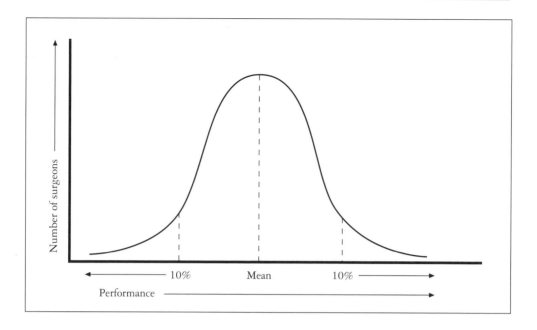

These surgeons cannot possibly see and treat all patients. Even if surgeons were equally good, about half would have below average results. Though there is a relationship between volume and outcomes, this is not linear but involves a threshold below which result are expected to be worse. Thus, good results from 'specialised' operations are not directly proportional to the volume of this specialised work done, but do depend on a threshold i.e. a minimum volume of such work, e.g. 7 to 10 colorectal operations a year constitute a minimum. Any number equal or above this has been calculated to be compatible with good operative results *(Taylor, I.)*. This has been shown to hold in other branches of surgery: The false positive rate for sentinel node biopsy in surgery for breast cancer, was found to be related to quantitative training, but did not improve further than a figure just below 10% after a threshold of thirty 'training' operations *(Bergkvist, L. et al.)*. When the volume increases above this threshold the results do not improve further significantly. A fair amount of work on the relationship of case volume to outcome has been carried out basing on results of oesophageal surgery, *(Mathews, H.R., Powell, D.J., McConkey, C.C.)*, *(Miller, J.D., Jain, M.K., de GARA, C.J.)* and also other major cancer surgery *(Begg, C.B., Cramer, L.D., Hoskins, W.J., Brennan, M.F.)*. Even this is not invariable. Individual surgeons working in small volume hospitals may, exceptionally, get good results *(Reasbeck, P.G.)*, though such small volume results have to be carefully scrutinised before they are used as valid argument. Moreover assessments may be problematic due to case mix and difficulties in accumulating a statistically acceptable volume even by 'busy' surgeons. A policy limiting operations to high volume centres may have profound implications on any health service. Statistical studies in U.K. indicate that an undiscriminating limit of 50 procedures per year for twelve common elective procedures would result in the exclusion of 40% of the surgical firms from performing such operations. Reducing the limit to 12 procedures would result in a 2% exclusion. This would have serious logistic consequences. Besides, relatively run-of-the-mill procedures, e.g. recurrent inguinal hernia repair, may not occur sufficiently frequently to reach the predetermined limit. Should such operations be all performed in specialized centres? The evidence supporting such a policy is not overwhelming. Perhaps more research is needed on the effects and implications of implementing such a policy *(Dobson, R.)*. One must also admit that most surgeons start their careers with low case volumes and only with time, dedication, sweat and blood do they achieve their excellence. Furthermore, outcomes are influenced by factors other then just volume. A clear historical example is the comparison of the results after 170 mastectomies performed by Billroth who reported an 82% recurrence rate and Halstead's 50 cases resulting in a 6% recurrence rate.

Surgeon	Volume	Outcome
Billroth	170 mastectomies	82% recurrences
Halstead	50 mastectomies	6% recurrences

More recently, a study on surgery for rectal carcinoma showed a five-fold difference in the risk of death within five years depending on the surgeon *(McArdle, C.S., Hole, E.)*. Morbidity followed the same pattern *(Lerut, T.)*. This is not surprising. The surgeon's expertise is definetely a prognostic factor following major surgery. Another factor influencing outcome is the infrastructure, which influences the quality of peri-operative treatment. Centralization may be an answer in relatively rare conditions. In more common conditions, high level facilities for post-operative care are not crucial. Dutch gastric cancer trials *(Bonnekamp, J.J., Hermans, J., Sasako, M.)*, showed that when general surgeons interact or are advised by specialist surgeons, their results equal those of their advisers. Appropriate training programmes for new techniques are equally helpful *(Martling, A.L. et al.)*. Thus transmission of expertise and training, which involves continuous medical education as well as audit, is bound to pay in improved standards and results.

A more structured approach to the teaching of surgical technical skills has been introduced in the last couple of decades. Workshops provide a uniform approach to basic tasks but there is no mechanism to build on this. Rasmussen theorises that the first step in practical learning systems is the acquisition of skills, as a first step, which can be learned before the full theoretical knowledge required for their practical application is assimilated, but only applying certain rules. This is another application of Aristotelian practical thinking, described in an earlier chapter. At a second phase, these rules are elaborated with continued experience. The third phase is one of knowledge-based practice, the source of this knowledge being the best possible evidence obtained from theory, experience, as well as ethical and humanistic considerations *(Rasmussen, J., Lind, M.)*.

There are two types of measurable motor abilities: (i) Perceptual motor abilities involving coordination, dexterity and speed of manipulation. (ii) Physical proficiency abilities, which includes stamina, physical prowess etc. The attainment of technical skills involves three stages :

(a) cognition – understanding the task;

(b) integration –using efficient movements; the learner practices the task and eliminates error from the performance.

(c) automation –there is no need to think about each step, with consequent increase in speed, efficiency and precision. Once the operator has reached the stage of automation, he has to break the process down into its several steps to be able to teach it to others *(Fitts, A.M., Posner, M.I.)*.

The above model resulted from research using very simple tasks. It may or may not strictly apply to complex motor skills involved in operative surgery.

It seems that technical skills can be acquired in an artificial 'trainer' environment away from the operating theatre. Actual operating, however, cannot be discounted as a teaching method. Learning curves should be controlled by automatic self-initiated feedback from tutors. This is applicable to CME as well as to basic and higher surgical training *(Hall, J.C.)*.

Decision making is a higher intellectual function, which cannot be divorced from the manual skills in attaining good surgical performance. Both these aspects of surgical training should form part of C.M.E. and C.P.D. (Continuous Professional Development) programmes *(Hamdorf, J.M., Hall, J.C.)*. In the process of reaching surgical maturity one not only learns what operation to do and how to do it, but also when to do it, when not to do it and when to call for help.

Learning from Unexpected Clinical Situations

When confronted with an unexpected scenario, clinicians react positively in two stages: The immediate 'in-practice' reaction is to apply present and past experiences on unfamiliar events to the current problem. Later on one reflects 'on-practice', reflecting on what happened, the causes that led to the unexpected event, on the effectiveness or appropriateness of the solutions adopted, outcomes and on one's future attitudes *(Schon, D.A.)*. This, together with discussions with peers and searches for published literature on the specific problem, help in improving one's competence, knowledge, skills and attitudes.

Super-specialisation

The concept of super-specialisation is often poorly understood and even more badly applied. The commonplace reasoning amongst its strong supporters follows the logic of the industrial assembly line, where reduction in repertoire enhances practice and efficiency. The corollary of assembly line logic i.e. that workers who do fewer repetitive jobs are easy to train and are therefore 'cheap', is conveniently forgotten.

As a result of these all too readily accepted concepts, surgical repertoire is steadily contracting, at the expense of patients worldwide. One can consider the need for the generalist by looking at three scenarios: The first scenario is the metropolis, which is rightly considered as offering the most fertile ground for super-specialisation. Even here, though, patients do not present with a diagnostic label on their forehead and, besides this, the pathology may involve more than one system. Thus the wider repertoire of the generalist is certainly necessary for proper pigeon-holing and, perhaps, to provide more comprehensive treatment and continuity. The second scenario refers to peripheral hospitals including those in remote areas and small islands e.g. the islands off the coast of Scotland and elsewhere, as well aslow catchment regions e.g. Iceland. The need for a generalist in such circumstances is obvious. More obvious still is the need for generalist postgraduate training of clinicians who intend to practice in third world countries. Concentrating on super-specialisation in this scenario will certainly lead to increased morbidity and mortality *(Loefler, I.J.P.)*. The general surgeon is far from an extinct breed and he needs organised continuous medical education as much as and even more than others. In fact, one measure that has been proposed to help to solve the present critical staffing problem in the British NHS is a new form of specialist training to equip surgeons and physicians with multispecialty skills. This constitutes a welcome reversal of attitudes *(Dowie, R., Langman, M.)*.

Training in Pre-hospital Trauma Care

The need for training in and the development of, a specialised field, is sometimes dictated by social developments. Pre-hospital trauma care, especially in respect to road traffic accidents is a clear example of this.

Every day 3000 people die and 30,000 are seriously injured worldwide. This exceeds the mortality from malaria *(Murray, C.J.L., Lopez, A.D.)*. All prediction indicate a worsening of this statistic with road traffic crashes moving from the 9th to the 3rd in the world burden of disease by 2020. The medical profession needs to address the problem by continuing to develop specialised training in pre-hospital trauma care and encouraging research on the subject, especially work which takes into account local conditions. The 'responsibility' aspect needs tackling: These accidents concern everybody, but unless a representative body is created to deal with the problem, with the minimum of bureaucracy, then there will be nobody to take the necessary action.

Women in Medicine

50% of medical students and house officers, as well as 7% of specialist registrars in UK are women *(Evans, J., Golcare, M.J., Lambert, T.W.)*. The principle of equality between males and females in medicine really means that they should have equal opportunities and not that they should be treated in an identical manner. This should not surprise anybody. Even within either sex, personalities are different and should be dealt with accordingly. The fact that women in medicine, especially in the course of further training and specialisation, encounter particular problems indicates the need to address this problem on a wide front. Flexible training and working conditions may constitute some of the answers. It would, however, imply complex legal, economic, organisational, and logistic changes, including an increase in 'manpower' allotment to units employing women to allow for this flexibility.

Medical Errors

It is wrong to think that the only good doctor is a perfect doctor. In Medicine, because of the very nature of the discipline itself, which is probabilistic, errors occur and are common. One must also admit that it is human to err without proposing this as a blanket excuse for all errors. Attempts to hide or bury this fact do not help the doctor - patient relationship in the medium and long term. The tendency towards transparency is hindered by the fear of litigation, fear of tarnishing the public's faith in their doctors and ethical arguments about reporting errors without the patient's consent *(Horton, R.)*. The principle of common good dictates that what is important is the lesson that we learn from admitting and analysing a mistake. To achieve this one needs support systems to give feedback on performance. This helps to plan and implement Continuing Medical Education and correct areas where results are below par. Audit is an important activity in this field. It involves the analysis of health care and is designed to improve its delivery. When gold standards in patient management have been determined by clinical research, then audit will establish how well these techniques are being applied to the clinical situation, with the intention of encouraging improved outcomes *(Williams, O.)*. The explicit training and re-training requirements applied, for example, to Minimally Invasive Surgery, should be applied to other fields to avoid poor results in newly adopted techniques loosely attributed to 'learning curves', and where results of properly conducted audit shows below-par returns. The enforcement of such procedures should be the competence of properly constituted bodies and should not necessarily depend on whistle-blowing reports from medical colleagues.

The Harvard Medical Practice Study reviewed 30,000 hospital admissions and found adverse events occurring in 3.7% of these. Over half of these were preventable and 13.6% of the latter figure resulted in death *(Berwick, D.M., Leape, L.L.)*. More recent figures from UK indicate that medical errors occur in 10% of hospital admissions. Even in this series, half of these are preventable and one third result in disability or death *(Vincent, C., Neale, G., Woloshynowych, M.)*. MEDMARX reports 105,603 medical errors in the USA in 2001. 2% of these occur in emergency departments, three quarters of which involve prescribing or administering drugs. Only 23% of these errors were intercepted before reaching the patient, compared with 39% in other departments *(MEDMARX)*. This is hardly surprising considering the pressure, urgency and time constraints in emergency departments.

Medical error may be classified by degree as: (a) Error with serious consequence. (b) No-harm event – though no harm resulted, there was potential for harm. (c) Near-miss i.e. Unwanted consequences were avoided because of planned or unplanned correction of the error *(Battles, J.B., Shea, C.E.)*. In addition error could be causally sub classified as follows:

Errors may result from systems failure, fatigue or through improper delegation to junior staff of work that necessitates more expertise. This may result in operative

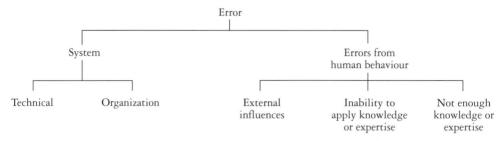

errors, prescribing errors, mistakes in carrying out medical procedures or in diagnosis. The converse is sometimes also true, in that errors and inefficiencies in care may in part be related to the excessive time spent by junior staff on non-clinical activities requiring a low level of skill. This effect is aggravated by the trend towards the reduction of working hours. Adequate reorganization of this aspect would increase the proportion of time dedicated to patient care. System shortcomings are more often responsible than errors arising from human behaviour *(Reason, J.)*. Operative errors may be reduced if fewer operations are performed during the night, by better surgical training, and by employing more experienced specialists to cover on-take hours. This does not necessarily mean that the solution is the introduction of consultant-based systems, which would itself generate serious disadvantages e.g. operations performed by exhausted consultants, low morale, early retirement. The logistics as well as the training of the on-duty staff should be adequate and their remuneration proportionate to the level of expertise expected of them. A computer linked pharmacology system, perhaps one organised on a national level, would help to reduce prescribing errors. Mishaps during medical procedures would surely diminish with better practical training programmes. Better training in surgical thinking, together with wider use of diagnostic algorithms and protocols should improve diagnostic accuracy if one is aware of the limitations of these aids. One would hope that with more investment in training and a national campaign to encourage the accurate and timely reporting of medical error especially by minimising the presently prevalent blame culture from our system, adverse events would diminish *(Alberti, K.G.M.M.)*. Safer systems of care and promoting instruction in surgical thinking, including clinical problem solving should pay dividends. This includes evidence-based decision making but also many other aspects of clinical problem solving and decision making e.g. Aristotelian practical reasoning. The ready availability of evidence (knowledge) is essential for this process. One must integrate research, education, library facilities and audit, thereby underlining the importance of education and research while, at the same time, encouraging the sharing of good ideas and practice. Because of the close relationship of post-graduate medical education and the delivery of medical care by health service employed trainees, compulsory and voluntary reporting of error is even more important. Root cause analysis of such reports would be invaluable to correct and improve educational and organizational systems.

Though self regulation has its benefits, it may not suffice. This is also evident in non-medical fields. There is a need for a change in culture and in attitudes, with the development of an atmosphere where medical students, doctors and specialists can express their worries when in difficulty and obtain help, not punishment. The remedy for medical error is not exhortation, 'being careful' or punitive action. The answer is to alter the system of work so that it becomes very difficult to produce the error. Rather than getting rid of the bad apples and eliminating the negative tail of the performance curve, one should try to shift the whole curve towards the positive side. This may primarily involve re-designing of machinery, but besides this, every phase of human action in carrying out a task, e.g. data collection, clinical reasoning, clinical decision making and the skill of carrying out the task, can all be made safer. One accepts human fallibility as inevitable and improves systems and designs round that fact. There must be responsibility in delegation of tasks, keeping in mind the interests of present patients in addition to that of teaching and future patients. Audit, appraisal with feedback on performance, assessment and revalidation should be considered within this context, avoiding stigmatisation and sensationalism. Moves in this direction have been made in the form of performance league tables, or better still, control charts. Performance league tables are useful in comparing quality or outputs from different systems. They are, however, difficult to interpret and may be the cause of anxiety. Control charts are more useful in comparing outputs within the same system. Stigmatisation of poor performers is avoided and when poor performance is due to random variation or special causes, this is recognised. A systems approach to quality improvement is thereby encouraged (*Adab, P. et al.*).

Regulation

This has been defined as the sustained and focussed control exercised by a public agency over activities, which are valued by a community to achieve wider social goals.

In the last couple of decades, organisations including public ones have become more accountable and this necessarily leads to regulation. This has also the effect of removing the onus of unpleasant decisions and difficult issues from the politicians' court, at least on paper. The setting up of regulatory bodies also strengthens the central government's control of such organisations including health services *(Walshe, K.)*.

Regulatory bodies may adopt different proportions of two possible paradigms in the course of their work i.e. the deterrence paradigm (assuming that the regulated bodies are intrinsically self-interested), or the compliance paradigm (assuming that these are intrinsically goody-goodies). The relative proportions of these two paradigms utilised may vary according to various influencing factors, which may not always be the most logical or just. Incentives and sanctions (the carrot and the whip) may both be necessary, but the degree and strength of these should be limited to the least effective doses. One should avoid a tug-of-war situation or an atmosphere of confrontation also by involving third parties e.g. patients, staff, representatives of medical industry, other professions etc., thus widening the field of view of the regulatory body. Lastly, regulatory bodies have to strike a fine balance between being sufficiently independent and at the same time being themselves accountable to those who appointed the and to the public.

Professionalism in Medicine

Professionalism in medicine in the U.K. was the product of the medical Royal Colleges in the early 1500's. In 1858, The Medical Act united the medical profession. The General Medical Council was instituted about 150 years ago to develop an ethical code, exercise auto-regulation and organise medical education.

Professionalism involves: (i) A high level of intellectual and technical expertise. (ii) Autonomy in the practice and regulation of the discipline. (iii) A social commitment *(Friedson, E.)*. It is a well known fact that undergraduate and postgraduate medical education can be psychologically very stressful and may have lasting effects on the lives of students and doctors. It is therefore important that teaching professional development should not be regarded as a natural consequence, but should rather be actively included in the medical curriculum. The key aims of professional development are: (1) To understand professionalism and the consequent responsibilities. (2) To instil the development of personal values, qualities attitudes and behaviour fundamental to health care. (3) To ensure the understanding, application of these qualities and willingness to develop and further professional identity *(Stephenson, A., Higgs, R., Sugarman, J.)*. This may help to reduce the incidence of 'casualties' and aberrations resulting from our present systems.

Patient-identifiable Data

At this point one cannot ignore the thorny problem of patient-identifiable data and informed consent in relation to the above. Compulsory anonymisation of data as well as informed consent from all patients, to allow the use of identifiable data for audit and every type of research, would render these methodologically unsound (systematic bias). This would render clinical governance impossible and would go against the public interest. Patients should be made aware that use of such data is not only of benefit to an anonymous 'public interest', but also helps to improve the management of their own disease. Involvement of legislators, professionals and international bodies may help to clarify the issue for the sake of progress in medical management *(Al-Shahi, R., Warlow, C.)*.

Audit, Continuous Improvement and Evaluation

Change does not always result in improvement, but any improvement requires change. Significant change results from changing systems, not changing within systems *(Berwick, D.M.)*. The aims must be ambitious, specific and must matter to society i.e. they should meet external needs. One learns from making changes, then reflects on the consequences of these changes. When trying to make improvements one does not necessarily need irrefutable evidence, but enough data to allow the next step in learning to be taken. This is an application of practical reasoning (vide Ch.1). Work and change which is non-consequential should not be undertaken. For improvement to occur, one must challenge the status quo continuously by actively testing changes, which promise improvement, on a small scale. The aim of audit is not to use deterrence to improve quality. The former would be application of the Theory of the Bad Apple, which implies that people must be made to care. The corollary of this theory would be that there are thresholds and standards above which one is safe from being labelled a 'bad apple'. Human nature being what it is, such floors rapidly tend to become ceilings. Statistical methods are used to detect divergent performance by comparing confidence intervals for a particular set-up with a benchmark, which reflects the average results for all cases undergoing the same procedure. Confidence intervals provide a convenient but not necessarily accurate way to express uncertainty in estimates of surgical performance. Different case-mix, severity and bias are not taken into account. To allow for these variants more elaborate statistical methods would be necessary *(van der Meulen, J.)*. Since the ultimate aim is to improve patient care, it is important to identify the biological and social determinants of risk. Only then can one pinpoint the difference in the clinical process that explain the divergent risk-adjusted outcomes *(Halm, F.A., Chassin, M.R.)*. Even these improved statistical methods to highlight the 'bad apple' may be only a small part of the improvement process.

The Theory of Continuous Improvement *(Berwick, D.M.)*, on the other hand, postulates that, without abandoning surveillance and discipline, supplier and customer in care should function as partners for continuous improvement. This requires leadership, good patient- doctor relationship, respect for the health worker and substantial investment.

Audit may be defined as the systematic and critical analysis of the quality of medical care, including the procedures used for diagnosis and treatment, the use of resources and the resulting outcome as well as the quality of life for the patient *(Department of*

Health: Working paper 6. 1989). Its aims are to identify ways for improving and maintaining the quality of care for patients, assist in medical education and training and optimise the use of available resources. Clinical audit should be an intrinsic part of patient care and also an intrinsic part of continuous education and adult learning. Ideally, it should be initiated and led by clinicians while it is facilitated and resourced by management, in a professional environment. It should be a confidential process, not to be used as an administrative punitive weapon. Just as the results of research are subject to error because of various types of bias, so are the results of audit. One clear example is 'gaming': The best way to obtain good results and favourable audit reports is to treat patients who did not need treatment in the first place!

One may describe a 4-stage audit cycle:

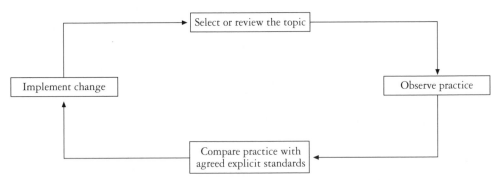

There are problems with the practical aspects of audit and quality assurance: Performance data is usually measured not on the basis of consistent performance but on that measured during a specific short period. Since these results do have consequences, resulting in either carrots or sticks, it is not surprising that a good amount of fiddling is common. What is thought to be measurable in, in fact, not measured accurately.

Though there is overlap between research and audit, these should be considered as two different entities: Medical research is a systematic investigation, which aims to increase the sum of knowledge and usually involves the testing of a hypothesis. It often involves random allocation into different groups and the occasional use of a placebo. Medical audit, is a systematic approach to peer review of medical care in order to identify and bring about, possible improvements. There is no random allocation or use of a placebo. Besides, whilst in medical research, strict selection criteria are applied before patients are entered into a study, there is no such selection when one carries out audit. Even when audit is applied to the assessment of different treatments for the same clinical problem, patients are allowed to choose freely their preferred therapy after adequate information *(Madden, A.)*.

The equivalent of audit in the educational process is termed 'evaluation'. It aims at local quality control of curricula and teaching methods. Because of its subjectivity to bias, its results can be rendered more reliable by increasing the number and levels of sources.

Clinical Governance

The concept was developed from that of 'corporate governance' which was established by the Cadbury Commission (1992) for the proper management of companies. Through this framework, health services commit themselves to a continuous improvement in the quality of their services and safeguarding of their standards of care, by creating an environment in which clinical excellence will flourish. Clinical decision making merges into the areas of organisation and management. One must do the right things in addition to doing things right *(Donaldson, L.J., Muir Gray, J.A.)*. One has to admit that the doctor-manager relationship is regarded less favourably by doctors than by managers *(Davies, H.T.O. et al.)*. It is possible to improve this state of affairs by the introduction of basic management techniques as part of the medical curriculum, joint post-graduate training programmes for both doctors and managers fostering a common language and approach, and encouraging a multidisciplinary approach to management decisions. The common ground is that clinicians and administrators at every level all work for the benefit of patients.

Quality

Quality is doing the right things to the right people at the right time and getting this right first time. Quality of care involves many aspects, including the technical quality of care, which is strongly influenced by organisational factors (Clinical governance), the quality of communication e.g. the doctor - patient relationship and patient information, patient compliance and the amenities i.e. the hotel aspects, for care. Improvement of quality requires good leadership, staff empowerment, teamwork, prevention rather than correction of adverse outcomes, as well as analysing, simplifying and improving processes that have a strong social commitment. Quality is central to the responsibilities of Health Organizations and individual professionals. The goal should be to meet national standards and where relevant, follow national guidelines. Clinical management, as in other fields, requires quantification, a realisation that every action carries its cost implication and that people will modify their behaviour to conform to protocols if they have respect for them.

Continuous Medical Education and Continuing Professional Development

Continuous Medical Education (CME) has been defined as 'any and all ways by which doctors learn after the formal completion of their training' *(Davies, D.)*. This definition seems, to me, rather restrictive and also contradictory since the process assumes that formal medical training should never end. It has been already pointed out that medical 'knowledge' is in a continuous state of flux. This is hardly something related to modern technology. Osler clearly recognised that 'from Hippocrates to Hunter the treatment of disease has been one long traffic in hypothesis' (Chapter on Surgical Treatment). One could clearly add 'and ever since' to this statement. As a result of this a medical student cannot bracket himself off from updating himself - hence Continuous Medical Education - during his student days, even from his very first encounter with medical training in its wider sense. Even at undergraduate level, topics are visited and revisited, with different emphasis and including recent advances. Undergraduate and postgraduate education should follow an integrated, though not homogenous, design. CME helps in the generation, appreciation, diffusion, critical appraisal and utilization of new knowledge at all levels, leading to better patient care *(Bennett, N.L. et al.)*. It is primarily teacher driven and is not in itself directed towards professional development. Doctors need more than update their knowledge. They also need to improve and sharpen their various skills, including communication, new technologies etc. This has been labelled as 'Continuing Professional Development' (C.P.D.), which involves both professional learning and personal growth. This is primarily learner centred and subjective and only indirectly affects public health. The methods used may involve the use of learning portfolios that are flexible, practical and accountable. Industry sponsored CME is, however, suspect. If unchecked it may be abused for marketing purposes.

Besides the flux of basic data, CME is affected by other forces, such as social and demographic ones including the globalisation of health, availability of data on patients, incorporation of principles of adult education, evidence based medicine, financial and public accountability and technological advances. On the negative side of the issue one has to include problems of funding and doctors' time (see Surgical Treatment page 4) and also different languages, training and cultures, and variation of economic status and healthcare deliveries on a global level *(Towle, A.)*. The information gap between rich and poor, between and within countries, is widening. However the electronics revolution, which is one of the causes of this, has the potential to reverse this trend, since it provides a cheaper and faster means of communication and information flow. Publishers in rich countries could contribute by providing medical educational material to developing countries for free, in the process creating a market for such information flow. This could be reciprocated by scientists in developing countries, with information flowing in all directions *(Godlee, F.)*. There may also be a corollary to this in an increased demand for the technology that usually accompanies such information and training. The weakness of this concept lies in the low research capacity of developing countries. It requires a genuine and persistent international effort to break this vicious cycle to create an information market and encourage health equity in such countries. There have been successful attempts at this type of international cooperation, e.g. research on malaria. Developing countries should behave and be allowed to behave, as partners in research and not as recipients of 'charity', or worse still, material for research. Investment in research capacity is more profitably done in the middle or long-term e.g. funding bodies to train researchers.

Knowledge Translation

Knowledge translation focuses on health outcomes and changing behaviour set in a practical environment *(Davies, D., Evans, M. et al.)*. By selecting evidence and producing aids and tools for their diffusion (e.g. clinical flowcharts, algorithms, guidelines, academic detailing and reminders) to all those involved in the healthcare process, including patients and policy makers, it is probably effective in narrowing the divide between evidence, clinical practice and patient adoption and compliance.

Technological Advances and CME

Recent technological advances used in CME include computer based learning methods e.g. CD ROM, internet access to medical literature for students, doctors, specialists and the public, distance learning e.g. satellite television for educational purposes or for practice e.g. teleradiology or telemedicine in general, virtual reality technology for surgeons and interventional radiologists. Several computerised programmes for updating clinical competence are already in use world-wide *(Parboosingh, J.)*. These include advanced multimedia computerised technology e.g. virtual reality technology to help train surgeons in invasive and laparoscopic procedures as well as TURP *(Satava, R.M., Jones, S.B.)*. Netprints and the National Electronic Library for Health have been set up in an attempt to harness internet technology to deal with the information overload, but may, paradoxically, exacerbate the problem due to sheer volume. These advances in communication and information technology bring new opportunities and challenges to medical education requiring new strategies in the design of curricula. Information technology skills have become essential in a profession highly dependent on electronic information, even though medical education leans heavily on practical training at the bedside. Campus networks help students select what to consume from the rivers of data provided on internet. The increase in student numbers and practical communication problems resulting from the posting of students at district hospitals for longish periods provoked the development of the 'virtual campus'. Its use is not limited to administration but is used in teaching especially as structured programmes of problem-based learning. At Guy's, King's and St. Thomas' School of Medicine this development has been found useful for flexible group work facilitated by a tutor. These technologies help to tailor learning to the individual patient and the teaching can be provided by the foremost experts on particular subjects. The student can time himself, repeat and even test himself at will. Computer-assisted learning facilitates the teaching of problem-oriented clinical reasoning and is useful for topics involving images or sounds e.g.anatomy, histopathology, endoscopy and auscultation signs. Interactive virtual-reality simulations more recently combined with tactile feedback (haptics), has been used effectively for teaching practical procedures e.g. catheterisation, TURP, laparoscopy and angioplasty. Computerised mannequins have been used to teach semeiotics and to simulate clinical and therapeutic scenarios. There are dangers in this technological expansion: The less affluent students and even countries could be handicapped and the demarcation between what is known and what can be retrieved from the web can become hazy. Medical educators have to establish what a clinician needs to know and what information is best accessed with evidence-based tools. With such rapid technological expansion one must apply cost-benefit considerations and make provision for teaching the teachers *(Ward, J.P.T. et al.)*.

Assessment of Clinical Competence

Postgraduate medical training in the past century has been influenced by the principles introduced by Osler, Welch and Halstead. In North America this is practiced through fixed period residency training which has not changed in essence during the last forty years. In a study assessing the outcomes of such training of neurosurgeons in the USA, programme directors doubted the competence of a small percentage of trainees who had just completed such training programmes but were due to be certified. Furthermore 10% of the trainees themselves had serious doubts about their competence *(Bosc, C.)*. Though postgraduate training in Europe is more articulated and in a sense more competence-based, the assessment of competence has not been effectively standardised in the different countries and is far from perfect. Despite EU legislation there have been several instances when certification in a speciality in one EU country has been refused acknowlegement in another. One needs improved reliable methods of performance assessment and systematic, possibly standardised approaches to re-licencure.

In hospital medicine, there are three types of controls on clinical competence;
(a) Revalidation, recertification and re-accreditation – where the 'bad apples' whose standards fall below accepted levels are identified.
(b) The contract review or negotiation – where the management, perhaps using output and audit results, pursues the interests and goals of the employer, while the clinician pushes his professional and developmental needs.
(c) Mentoring or Professional review – a reflective, non-judgemental, confidential meeting between the clinician and a trusted person, involving exchange of ideas, advice and plans but not negotiations *(Bulstrode, C., Hunt, V.)*.
The outcomes of such meetings or methods of control may be synergistic but should be considered as distinct.

Appraisal, Recertification and Revalidation

Appraisal is a structured process of facilitated self reflection, allowing a comprehensive assessment of one's strengths and areas requiring improvement, aiding insight as part of the learning cycle. A form of appraisal and assessment for surgeons was introduced by Zoroaster in Persia over two and a half millennia ago *(Garrison, F.H.)*. The association between appraisal and improved outcomes *(West, M.A.)* seems to depend on the sophistication of the appraisal process. Appraisal could provide the elusive bond between clinicians and managers because they both share the same goal of improved outcomes.

Though the concept of recertification or revalidation is a spinous one, which encounters expected resistance, a programme of continuous recertification (as opposed to sporadic assessments) may be an effective way of maintaining professional knowledge and performance. It is highly probable that consultants will have to accept some form of regular recertification or revalidation and it is just as well that they contribute to devise simple, effective and fair methods of doing this. Revalidation systems in UK seem to be developing towards five successive appraisals. Appraisal and revalidation must be centred on learning and based on the learner to result in improved levels of care. These methods of lifelong learning, should complement and not replace present initiatives with the same objective. This could be done by providing doctors with online learning resources based on best available evidence e.g. BMJ learning, combining systematic audit of practice data and documented evidence of continuous learning. Computer programmes could be used to monitor doctors' performance, patient outcomes, cost-benefit considerations, peer reviews and perhaps patient's views on doctors' attitudes including communication skills. There are several admirable initiatives, e.g. the one by The Royal College of Physicians and Surgeons of Canada, but none are sufficiently comprehensive. The process must include certain essential requirements: It should include a wide range of learning resources that can be adopted for the various styles of learning. Learners must be guided to the use of these resources and their needs identified and resolved. Subsequently their efforts are recorded and assessed.

It is unfortunate that it needed adverse press on reported cases of professional negligence, followed by public and political concern (not always guided by good knowledge) to prod the Colleges to take a lead in such innovations in self regulation. Such initiatives may contribute to revitalise the necessary trust and respect in the doctor - patient relationship. It would be a step forward if in the future such initiatives are ingrained in the statutes and structures of our regulatory bodies and colleges so that the required reforms will be less painful.

Recertification programmes lead to pressure on doctors which may result, also, in undesirable side effects e.g. the growth of self-designated 'certifying boards' of varying reliability, the development of alternative attributes of competence e.g. accreditation - which adds to the general confusion, the proliferation of programmes which help clinicians to pass recertification exams and not quite aimed in improving clinical practice. Finally 'attending' such updating programmes is not synonymous with 'attention' to the teaching delivered.

Of course, any continuous educational process has to be regularly evaluated in all its stages i.e. the instructional quality, learner's perception, the learning behaviours, eventual competence of the learner and finally, the product. The evaluating methods to be used can be multiple but may include: learner satisfaction questionnaire, intrinsic motivation questionnaire, process evaluation records, and outcome assessment.

Scholarship

Scholarship involves four overlapping components: (i) Discovery (ii) Integration (iii) Application and (iv) Teaching *(Boyer, E.L.)*. Of these, integration has received the least attention. This involves making connections across disciplines and placing specialities in a larger context of knowledge. Though such knowledge is too vast for any person to absorb, there is a distinct need to bring diverse fields more closely together so as to get their data into perspective and give new insights into this knowledge. Medicine will thus move from the margins to the mainstream of academia *(Dauphinee, D. et al.)*. Research in life sciences is directed at improving health as an ultimate goal. However most advances result from breakthroughs in other fields e.g. MRI, Positron emission tomography, fibreoptics etc. It is obvious that cross-pollination between disciplines improves the chances of problem solving. The scholarship of integration is the intellectual effort which helps to improve medical education in its entire spectrum, improve communication with the community, raise the efficiency of processes in any practical sciences, and ensure quality of research and maintainance of competence. The scholarship of application involves the translation of fundamental knowledge into practical use, rendering it useful, testable and reproducible.

Undergraduate and probably also postgraduate education must include training in techniques and strategies of interprofessional collaboration in its wider sense. Doctors need training in communication, with their patients, with other doctors and with other professionals. This should include coaching in thinking and problem-solving (this is, after all the scope of this work), training in sustained attention, coaching as groups rather than as individuals, and opportunities to plan and initiate changes in clinical attitudes, record results and assess advantages or otherwise of these changes. Different types of assessments e.g. essay questions, MCQ's, traditional clinical and viva voce exams, as well as computer-based case simulation and standardised patient exams, measure different areas of competence. It is therefore logical to use multiple modalities in assessments *(Edelstein, R.A.)*.

Surgical Training

There is an increasing public demand for accountability of clinicians in order to protect the public. In addition to this, a general awareness has developed amongst doctors, especially surgeons, that it is important to recognise deficiencies in competence and technique, which would allow early and appropriate correction, or in extreme cases, advice to pursue an alternative career. There is an obvious need for reproducible and valid checks on the different aspects of clinical, especially surgical, competence.

The training curriculum, methods for evaluating trainees and assessment of the programme are all interdependent. The reduction in clinical exposure time of surgical trainees is worrying. Before the Calman reforms and the European Working Time Directive, a trainee worked about 30,000 hours between becoming a Senior House Officer and getting a consultant post. This exposure period has now fallen to 8,000 hours *(Phillip, H. et al.)* and is expected to contract further to 6000 hours i.e. one fifth of the time! This cannot be entirely compensated by an increased intensity or efficiency of training methods. There is also a serious regress in continuity of care. Surgical training must be recognised as a priority and incentivised. The introduction of courses in basic surgical skills by the Colleges was a welcome innovation in surgical training. Animals have been used for this. However animal substitutes, such as jigs and bench models, which could be realistic, or in the form of a series of structured tasks e.g. peg transfers or pattern cutting, may be adequate substitutes. They can even be applied for training as well as assessment in minimal access surgery. The University of Toronto has developed the Objective Structured Assessment of Technical Skills (OSATS): While trainees perform operative tasks on simulation models, they are evaluated by trained surgeon observers, using structured checklists and global ratings *(Matsumoto, E.D., Reznick, R.K.)*.

Virtual reality is defined as a collection of technologies which allow efficient interaction with 3D computerised databases in real time using one's natural senses and skills. The developments in the internet and e-learning led to the diffusion of simulation techniques, interactive 3D images and structured courseware applied in general surgery, orthopaedics, anaesthesia, emergency medicine, cardiology and even psychiatry. The considerable expense of surgical training, curtailed working hours and shortened training programmes are incentives for the development and application of these technologies. A good proportion of surgical technique is thus acquired outside the operating theatre. The applications, even at present, are numerous: Veniipuncture, therapeutic gastroscopy, ERCP, colonoscopy, lumbar puncture and brain ventricular taps. Virtual reality computer simulation has been successfully used for surgical training of Trans-urethral resection of the prostate, *(Briggs, T.P., McDonald, D., Gardner, J.E., Mundy, A.R.)* and minimal access surgery where various aids have been developed e.g. the minimally invasive surgery trainer –virtual reality system (MIST-VR), for assessment of endoscopic manipulative competence – Advanced Dundee Endoscopic Psychomotor Tester (ADEPT). These methods have a disadvantage with immediate feedback but are economical on teaching manpower *(Hamdorf, J.M. and Hall, J.C.)*. Each task can be programmed to deliver varying degrees of difficulty. The trainee's performance can be saved for scrutiny by the supervisor or for statistical analysis. This training has been shown to lead to equivalent performance in the operating theatre *(Gallagher, G.)*. Virtual reality systems are used routinely in some centres ,to plan operations e.g. maxillo-facial and other plastics operations. Another use of this technology is for the objective assessment of clinical skills and assessment of aptitude for surgical work. One is not hereby proposing total reliance for these aims on this technology. The influence of virtual reality and simulation in enhancing surgical training will be directly proportional to the increase in computer power and availability *(Gorman, P.J., Meier, A.H., Rawn, C., Krummel, T.M.)*. Robotic procedures, such as the da Vinci system has been used for laparoscopic work, CABG and other vascular surgical procedures. In the future one can predict the application of virtual reality technology to procedures using micro-robots or nano-robots controlled by skilled operators.

Despite the well-known difficulties, the development of reliable and valid methods of assessment in the operating theatre environment, are still highly desirable. One has to admit that present-day assessment in the operating theatre is not that reliable because of the tense atmosphere, the widely varying independence afforded to the trainees, the variations of difficulty grade even of specified operations and the standardisation of assessment. Further research into this aspect of training is clearly necessary. Efforts to deliver better training and assessment should not be done defensively in response to controversies, but rather as a positive action for the common good.

Conclusion
It is now established that CME can improve health care - the improved Gotland suicide rate study is one example *(Rutz, W., von Knorring, I., Walender, J.)*. This improvement in quality of care through CME can be achieved only if doctors are psychologically at their best. Doctors should be as psychologically healthy as they would like their patients to be. The two factors, which have a major influence on doctors' wellbeing, are the doctors' personal values and choices, e.g. family, friends, religion, philosophical outlook, and the control they have over their external work environment, e.g. their influence over decision making, autonomy and in planning their work output. The common goal of improving health care on a global level should help to overcome the above mentioned difficulties if enough enthusiasm and dedication are injected into our trainees and colleagues. It is one path in our efforts to reduce the much greater difficulties that our patients have to face. Hopefully it will bring us nearer to Boerhaave's limit of scientific certainty, which with equal certainty, we shall never reach.

Chapter 6

Consuming Surgical Research

Quotation:
  R. Oppenheimer (1904 – 1967): 'Both men of science and men of art live at the edge of mystery, surrounded by it; both always, as the measure of their creation, have had to do with the harmonization of what is new with what is familiar, with the balance between novelty and synthesis, with the struggle to make partial order in total chaos.'

Introduction

The practising doctor is subjected to all sorts of pressures 'to move with the times'. The pharmaceutical industry bombards him with glossy publications written in pseudo-scientific terms: he may even be invited to sponsored talks, conferences and 'drug-do's; (in this respect the Royal College of Physicians has issued clear updated guidelines. These, and an account of rules that are applied in different countries have been published by *McGuaran, A.*), patients may demand certain forms of treatment, and he may harbour a natural desire to 'keep up with the Jones'. The public, and to some extent the profession, share an expectation that an everlasting, disease-free life is just round the corner.

The only way that a practitioner can maintain a balanced outlook, distinguishing between a real advance and a passing fashion, is by accepting a commitment to continuing education. This should aim at providing the surgeon or student with the necessary knowledge and skills to make appropriate decisions in line with present day practice. 'External clinical evidence', in the form of published research can inform, but never replace individual clinical expertise. It is the latter, which will allow a decision of the applicability of the research results to the individual patient and how it can be integrated into a management strategy.

Problems

There are problems in this continuous accumulation of an ever-increasing body of information about the practice of surgery. This is due to:

(i) Increasing surgical progress.
(ii) Increasing volume of information presented in journals, promotional material and surgical meetings. The involvement of commercial organisations in this respect, gives rise to concern in that the surgeon's (or student's) limited 'knowledge bank' may be invaded by information which may not represent an unbiased view of current surgical thought. The problem of sheer volume of

research information is accentuated by the introduction of registration of clinical trials at their inception, and the unification of such registers *(Tonks, A.)*. About 10,000 new RCT's are included in Medline every year. 350,000 have been identified by the Cochrane collaboration. A further increase in volume has resulted from the introduction of netprints, where scientific work may be published before peer review, in the same way as the presentation of scientific results at meetings or conferences. One such electronic archive is PubMedCentral, intended as a barrier-free repository of life sciences research reports and supporting research. This practice has been accepted in other scientific disciplines e.g. high-energy physics. The scope of these developments is transparency and openness of the clinical research process, and this is both desirable and laudable. It will, however, increase the load of external clinical evidence *(Delamothe, T., Smith, R., Keller, M.A. and Witsher, B.)*. This 'evidence' is presented in various forms, involving narrative, qualitative information, quantitative data or statistical models. The problem of too much information is not limited to medicine, but even in other aspects of life this has adverse effects: Vital intelligence information before the 11th September was ignored because it was so diluted by information overload. Modern information technology provides us with powerful tools with which to filter useful information from a large volume of information *(Kostoff, R.)*. These methods involve information retrieval, infrastructure identification, literature-based discovery of new concepts and relationships, identification of main themes, their relationship and their relevance and effect on clinical practice. All this needs training, time and expertise.

(iii) The necessity to assimilate information which is only tangentially related, but which may be profitably applied to surgery.

The time required to keep abreast of all medical advances has been estimated as what it takes to read 19 to 20 articles per day, daily *(Shaneyfelt, T.)*, while the estimated time really available is more like an hour a week or less *(de Dombal, F.T.)*. It is obvious that clinicians have to be trained in information-seeking skills and also critical appraisal in selecting potentially useful articles. One must however, have a correct understanding of the relationship between training in critical appraisal and improvement in clinical decision making. Literature on this relationship is scarce, but seems to indicate a direct relationship between these two capabilities *(Neville, A.J. et al.)*.

Publications

Most papers are presented in standard IMRAD format: Introduction (reason for the research), Methods (how the research was done and results analysed), Results (what was concluded) and Discussion (what the results mean). The discussion should also be structured and should not be the most arbitrary and most unscientific part of the paper. Certain essential points have to be clearly presented i.e. the authors' particulars, the introduction including the scientific basis for the study, informed consent and data collection forms, the study design, eligibility and exclusion criteria, the method including details of treatment in each study arm, side effects of treatment and any modifications, the required monitoring during treatment and follow-up, evaluation of outcomes and the references. One should:

(i)   Clearly re-state the research findings

(ii)   Discuss the strengths and weaknesses of the study without bias.

(iii)   Compare the strengths, weaknesses and results with those of other studies, pointing out and explaining the differences with minimal speculation.

(iv)   Explain the findings and discuss their implications.

(v)   Discuss unanswered questions and suggest future research in the field *(Smith, R.).*

(vi)   When evaluating outcomes, one may refer to survival, freedom from disease recurrence or progression, objective evaluation of change in pathological process e.g. tumour size, improvement in symptoms, quality of life or side effect of the intervention.

(vii)   References must be verified against the original documents. This rule has been standard practice for ages amongst historians. It is entirely practical to adhere to these standards. Such information can be downloaded from Medline with the bibliographic aids e.g. Endnote, ensuring accuracy of reference lists *(Siebers, R., Holt, S.).*

Reporting in medical journals has evolved from descriptive case reports to describing and naming syndromes, to reports on treatments, to randomised controlled trials and systematic reviews. The latest development is a shift from describing the phenotype to pinpointing the relevant genetic defect.

One can assess the quality of a paper by estimating the clarity and importance of the question, correctness of the method, validity and applicability of the conclusion and effectiveness of communication. However, the decision whether to continue reading a paper, usually depends on the section on design and methods. The criteria and considerations, which can be used for efficient consumption of research, are equally useful when considering which research to fund or which research papers merit publishing.

Scientific publications are often full of reports of experimental observations that achieve status because they have been carried out by the latest and most-expensive techniques and not because they are designed to test some particularly interesting scientific idea or postulate. As a consequence scientific literature is overwhelmed by mere reportage of observations that are published as such, without organic relationship to precisely formulated hypothesis. Such observations are scientifically meaningless. Furthermore, only 6% of drug advertising material is supported by evidence *(Tuffs, A.)*.

The surgeon's mind functions like an information system of limited channel capacity (training can only alter this very marginally), which is overloaded with information that is largely irrelevant and sometimes misleading.

The Clinician's Reaction

The possible reactions to this may be:

(a) ignoring new developments - the surgeon continues to practice his profession up to the standards when he stopped taking in new data,

(b) uncritical evaluation and adoption of research results and of new techniques e.g. taking a new therapeutic technique from a 'meeting' may be dangerous. A result is more likely to be uncritically accepted as a 'fact', and repeated ad infinitum if it is quantified, than if it is not quantified *(Black, N.)*. It seems that the printing of a number is accepted as a guarantee of accuracy without prompting an in-depth inquiry into sources, methods etc. One example: 'Malta has a 1 in 12 lifetime risk of developing breast cancer' (initially calculated on a 3 year statistic with potentially faulty sources, data and material). Another example is the widely accepted concept of Percentage Disability in medical certification. There are a number of volumes written on the subject which give reassuring numerical values for specific disabilities. The basis for the allocation of such definite percentages, which are actually just conventions, is quite suspect, especially because the various authorities do not always agree on the figures *(Mc Bride, E.D.)*, *(Griffiths, V.G.)*. The reason for the insistence on such definite numerical values is not their exactness, but the fact that they facilitate the work of insurance companies and Court Judges regarding claims for compensation. Applying present Maltese Law, the person's compensation amounts to his earnings lost as a result of the degree of disability. Using this apparently precise method, the life of a worker is worth a small percentage of the life of his boss! The introduction by the World Bank and W.H.O., of 'Disability Adjusted Life Years' (DALY), *(World Bank –World Development Report 1993)* similarly tries to fuse quality of life and length of life in a number. This is similarly flawed e.g. the life of a disabled person, or one who for some reason produces less and earns less, is undervalued.

Another example is the use of Impact Factors to assess the quality of research or the researcher. This is a numerical value obtained by dividing the number of times an article in a journal is cited, by the number of articles that could be cited, as published by the Science Citation Index. There is consensus of opinion that this value is scientifically meaningless and may be misleading in the above-mentioned assessment *(Seglen, P.O.)*. As an example, the top surgical journal has the same Impact Factor as the 25th ranking molecular biology journal, because articles by surgeons were less often cited by other researchers *(Burke, K.)*. Quality refers to the originality of subject thought and method. Excellent original research may have as its object rare diseases with little direct or indirect social effects. The matter is even more complex in that scientific quality of medical research and its social impact do not necessarily run parallel. To cite some examples: The research done on apoptosis over the last thirty years or so, is generally of very high quality, but has had little social impact. On the other hand, research on stoma appliances may not be scientifically impressive, but has had considerable social impact. For assessment to be fair, even in comparative rather than absolute terms, the rules have to be clear. Developing these rules is an even more difficult task when one includes social impact into the equation *(Smith, R.)*. We shall refer to this subject again when discussing systematic reviews and meta-analysis later on in this chapter.

(c) Denial: Through the consumption of reliable research one may come to realise that, however good one's overall performance has been, a particular practice has been proved as doubtful or potentially dangerous. This situation often results in the emotion of shame, which leads to denial and the raising of barriers to improvement *(Davidoff, F.)*. Thus, even reliable evidence may have the reverse effect to what is logically expected, if it dose not fall on the fertile soil of a strong character.

(d) Critical evaluation of new information so that one can separate the wheat from the chaff.

It is the latter reaction that this discussion will try to encourage.

Training for Consuming Research

Medical training should include methods, which help medical students to become good consumers of research i.e. that they can quickly evaluate which research project or findings they can utilise in their clinical practice or supporting services. Such training may be included with the present teaching of

1. Biostatistics (Concepts of measurement, statistical inference, types of study design).
2. Epidemiology esp. methods.
3. Public Health and Administration.

There are some practical measures that can reduce uncertainty in the interpretation of research: One should consider the results of a study in the context of all available research on the subject. Studies and especially their summaries must use precise language and logical as well as honest interpretation. Journals should show more willingness to publish admittedly uncertain results, so that authors would feel more free to admit the limits and uncertainties of their studies.

The recent history of science suggests that patterns of medical investigations and treatment will continue to change as a result of further discoveries, yet few of these changes will constitute so dramatic an advance as to require immediate and total acceptance. About 56 billion dollars per year are spent on health research, but only 10% of these are spent on diseases, which account for 90% of the world burden of disease *(Global forum for health research)*. Often, populations in poor countries are subjected to research which can only benefit richer countries because of the inherent costs of the application of the results of such research e.g. research on aids. It has been estimated that, in developing countries, 1% of the GPD should be directed to research *(Oumeish, O.Y.)*. Clinical (applied) research is playing second fiddle to its 'pure' counterpart, which, apart from being unfair, is probably, also, very unwise. Academic medicine should give clinical research, which will be increasingly backed by a molecular insight, more consideration *(Lindahl, S.)*. This must, however, be accompanied by mechanisms which assure practicality, applicability, consumption and absorption of its results.

Aim of Research

It is often assumed that a constant flow of knowledge from the research field to the bedside is critical to a high standard of health care. This idea is true as long as one realises that these two activities may well be carried out in different geographical regions with or without good communication. We may well be quite inefficient in putting these ideas into effect; for example, trauma, the most common killer before the age of 45 years, is not only poorly understood but scantily researched. It also commonly assumed that embarking on research is cost-effective. Even in general terms this is most unlikely since new knowledge and technology hardly ever decrease costs. One exception to this statement is research in preventive medicine.

Research is a procedure, or a sequence of activities consisting of selecting, observing, recording, comparing, analysing, classifying the phenomena and finally deriving appropriate inferences and perhaps integrations. There are two aspects of this:

(i)   reflections on a problem, (Plate 7)
(ii) action designed to investigate nature.

Plate 7

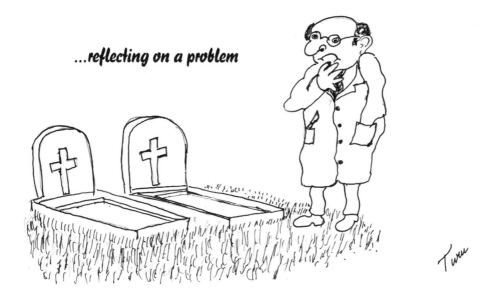

...*reflecting on a problem*

The pathways of scientific discovery may be shown graphically as follows:

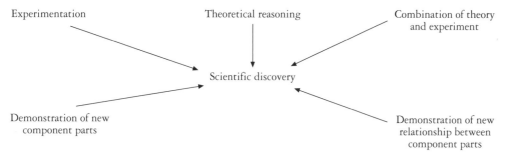

A scientific discovery consists of the demonstration of either a new component part or a new relationship between component parts. This can be achieved by experimental manipulation of the object of study, by theoretical reasoning, or most frequently, by combination of the two. Thus the use of recombinant human activated protein C in the treatment of severe sepsis could be postulated on theoretical grounds because: patients with severe sepsis have low levels of activated protein C; activated protein C inhibits activated factors V and VIII and therefore decreases the formation of thrombin; it also reduces the concentration of plasminogen activator inhibitor type 1 and therefore fibrinolysis and also reverses the procoagulant and inflammatory effect of sepsis. Experimentally it has been found to improve the clinical outcome in meningococcal septicaemia.

Medical research, in its wider sense, seeks a comprehension of the human being in health and disease. The position today about most diseases known to medicine is that pathogenesis is understood fully or partially, but the aetiology (i.e. the basic cause) remains obscure. This is the most significant single justification of medical research. It is justified by the value of its applications e.g. the application of the results of immunological research to transplant surgery, or of genetics to the prevention or early treatment of cancer. It may conceivably be justified by the intrinsic worth of this knowledge e.g. research in comparative anatomy or in determining the growth rate of different finger and toe nails *(Harre R)*. In practice, several situations may prompt a medical researcher to initiate a project:

1. Current knowledge does not satisfy a certain question or questions,

2. A phenomenon is observed which is not explained by current knowledge,

3. To test another researcher's hypothesis,

4. The development of new and better methods of analysis.

The medical researcher should take a utilitarian approach and design studies that take into account how and by whom the results will be used, since there have to be priorities in implementing research results. The Declaration of Helsinki states, amongst other things: 'Medical research is only justified if there is a reasonable likelihood that the population in which it is carried out stands to benefit from the results of the research.' *(World Medical Association)*. The application of these results involves a synthesis of the evidence, development of a clinical policy and application of this policy. There is a clear place for the clinical scientist, but he should be encouraged to produce work with clinical impact. How else would the taxpayer be convinced that his support is worthwhile? In return, careers in clinical science should be better structured and protected, and research quality assessed more scientifically. Having said this, one must admit that research into conditions or situations which are, at face value, rare or narrow fields, will not only help the patients suffering from these rare conditions (these patients have a right to the best possible management), but may throw light on more common diseases. Examples of this abound: Williams Syndrome (first described by Fanconi in Switzerland) is a rare condition (1 in 10,000 to 1 in 50,000 births in different series) effecting elastin fibres. The discovery of the genetic defect in chromosome 7q, may well lead to advances in other more common diseases involving elastin. Optimising cardiac output and oxygen delivery prior to elective operations was originally worked out for open cardiac surgery but promises dramatic reduction in mortality in trauma, emergency surgery and even elective major general surgical cases. Research into rare systemic infections with Mycobacterium avium intracellulare led to a discovery of a gene defect effecting gamma receptor interferon which results in the inability to handle, other more common intra cellular pathogens e.g. Salmonella, Listeria and Leishmania. More tangibly, the general mortality in children below the age of five years has decreased by 15% over the last couple of decades. This cannot all be attributed to the effects of research. Better nutrition, hydration and immunisation have certainly played a part. Research is however, involved in quantifying problems, pointing out strategies and assessing the effectiveness of these, including factors as those mentioned above. In developing countries the effects of research have not been so marked. The way ahead would be for research to be directed to the particular problematics of the local conditions and to have more cooperation between researchers, health workers, policy makers and the various constituted bodies and groups.

In applying research evidence to the individual patient one has to consider the physiological and psychological peculiarities of the patient, the risk to the patient if the research evidence is not applied, the social, cultural or economical factors that might influence suitability or acceptability of the management and also the patient's wishes and informed consent. This is another application of the general principle of weighing advantages against disadvantages and setting priorities *(Sheldon, Guyatt, Haines)*.

Corporate Influence on Research

The limited possibilities of receiving support for their research from public funds, has driven clinical (and other) scientists to resort to industry as their only source of funding. Consequently, most of their efforts are necessarily directed to these 'industrially useful' commitments. Though such collaboration may be fruitful, it is a historical fact that the most important advances have resulted from curiosity-driven science and occasionally serendipity e.g. the discovery of penicillin by Fleming. In addition, there is a distinct possibility of a conflict of interests between the scientist and the funding industry, which insists on tangible and economically useful results. This may result in undue and distorting influence on the body of published evidence. There is good reason to be concerned that the objectivity of the researcher and the value of the research to society may be influenced by commercial interests. The genome project is just one example of this conflict and the compromised intellectual independence of researchers. Encroachment on intellectual independence is not limited to private funding by powerful economic groups. Government departments can be similarly invasive. The early scientific reports on Bovine Spongiform Encephalitis (B.S.E.) and Creutzfeldt-Jacob disease, were discouraged by the U.K. Ministry for Agriculture, Fisheries and Food as uncovered by the Phillips Enquiry *(Swales, J.D.)*. Political issues often take priority over scientific pursuits. Research, even utilitarian (need-driven) research, requires independence and stability. This can only happen when the funding body has no vested interest in the particular outcome.

Authors of research publications are required to disclose any financial ties with companies that manufacture products discussed in their papers. These ties are often, however, so extensive, that it would take too much space to disclose them fully in journals! *(Angell, M.)*. Furthermore such disclosures are not sufficient guarantee against bias.

The ties of clinical researchers to industry are not limited to grant supports, but may range from sponsored symposiums to direct financial interest. Introducing strict guidelines may well be an answer, even at the cost of loosing researchers to other centres where a more relaxed and tolerant regulation in this respect exists. These more 'liberal' institutions may themselves have running partnerships with the pharmaceutical or medical technology industry as a form of symbiosis. It is anachronistic that this more 'liberal' scenario rarely results in more liberty for the researcher's scientific endeavours. The reasons in favour of this surrender of academic independence include: (i) To facilitate technology transfer, i.e. easier passage from research results to the market and (ii) to obtain vital financial backup for the research. In fact, more research is done to test a technology rather than to develop it. In addition personal rewards and interests have little to do with technology transfer. It would be more ethical and efficient if any 'rewards' for consultations were to go into a common fund directed widely for the institution's research programmes, hoping that these common funds would be used with good sense, efficiency and equity. The disadvantages of such dependence are; (i) Skewing of research towards what is more profitable, which may not concur with what is more necessary. (ii) Possible interpretative bias of the results of research. (iii) Possible 'spiking' of unfavourable results. (iv) Threatening of researchers, interruption of trials and blocking of publications *(Greenberg, D.S.)*. (v) Possible distraction from the clinical researcher's other duties e.g. teaching. Legal clauses in the contract of partnership cannot guard completely against the above possibilities. Co-operation between industry and academia should not result in lowering of ethical standards or in the inoculation of the interests of shareholders in industry into the decision- making mechanism of the clinical researcher. It is undeniable that medical science has been heavily contaminated by corporate money.

One way out of this dilemma is to have a national independent body to oversee and grade research and its funding through a common financial pool. Other suggested solutions to the problem include the complete separation of academic research from corporate money and the creation of a university ombudsman who has enough power to be immune from government and corporate pressure and who can help researchers who find themselves under this type of pressure.

Types of Research and Experimental Analysis
(a) Basic research - i.e. discovery of new phenomena.
(b) Applied research - applying existing knowledge to new situations.

There is considerable overlap of these two subdivisions, but most surgical research is of the applied type, where basic scientific information is used to further our knowledge and skills in prevention, diagnosis and management of human disease. Applied research may be subdivided in two categories:

(i) Disease-oriented research e.g. the discovery of insulin.

(ii)Patient-oriented research. Clinical research falls into this category.

Workers involved with patient-oriented research are less frequently adequately funded when compared with basic researchers. One way to improve this situation is to allow intellectual-property protection by patenting the results of patient-oriented research. The royalty payments that would result at the time of commercial application of their discoveries could be directed at further patient-oriented research. It would also encourage the interaction between clinical and basic research, as well as biotechnology in that applied (clinical) research does not lag behind for lack of funding, thus limiting the application of the results of basic research *(Rees, J.)*.

We shall henceforth be dealing essentially with clinical research and we shall not refer to experimental work with laboratory animals. It is pertinent, however, to make a brief reference to the present unhealthy polarisation on the subject of animal research. One way to favour the cause of both animals and humans is to work on the classical three R's of animal research *(Russel, W.M.S., Burch, R.L.)*. These refer to replacement, reduction and refinement. Replacement means the use of any scientific method employing non-sentient material instead of conscious, living vertebrates. The problem is that such molecular, cell, tissue or organ models, are too simplified when compared with animals and humans in their integrity. By reduction one means the lowering of the number of animals needed to obtain information. This requires optimal panning of research methodology and statistical analysis. Refinement refers to the limitation in incidence and severity of inhumane procedures applied to animals. With the application of the three R's, the number of animal experiments has halved, while the number of animals used has been reduced by 90% in the past twenty years *(Editorial: The Lancet)*. The use of genetic models for human disease, though complex, has the potential to reduce these numbers even further. Anachronistically however, this may also have the effect of increasing the use of higher animals, because biologically based compounds targeting human molecules may be only tested on such animals.

Clinical experimentation is, essentially, a comparison between the relative effectiveness of two or more forms of therapy. These studies may take two forms:

(a) Retrospective studies

(b)Prospective studies - these may be prophylactic or therapeutic.

In retrospective studies, the results of a particular treatment are compared with that obtained by another treatment, administered previously over a period of time. There may be bias in this method, in that one or more factors which may affect response, may vary in the two groups. Thus the results as best tentative, at worst misleading.

Prospective studies utilise simultaneous comparisons of treatments where these are allocated to two or more groups entirely at random. Randomisation was accepted as the basis of controlled clinical trials following the MRC Streptomycin trial in 1948. Patients are allocated to an 'experimental' and a 'control' group. The former are given the new treatment while the latter are given the 'old' or established treatment or else a dummy. Omission of controls might lead to excessive optimism in the interpretation of results *(Cuschieri, A., Baker, P.R.).*

Methods of Clinical Research

The methods used are designed to reach the ultimate aim of research that is, arriving to a conclusion from the hypothesis:

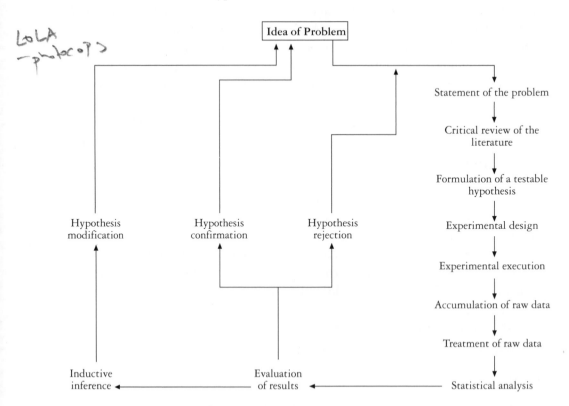

The research worker must acquire the ability to recognise a problem and analyse its various aspects so as to formulate a logical working hypothesis that might explain it. He then chooses the most effective available methods to test this hypothesis. An appropriate statistical design is essential so that results can be analysed to give meaningful data and therefore valid conclusions. There must be an adequate number of patients to detect a real difference between the two forms of treatment, if such a difference exists. Random allocation of patients ensures that the distribution of variables between the two groups is as 'equal' as possible.

When a new approach to treatment is deemed technically feasible and suitable for human trials, the process goes through three phases: In the first phase, a study is performed on a small number of patients and the problems inherent in the study are identified. In the second phase, a larger number of patients are included and the potential efficacy of the treatment under study assessed. In the third and final phase one compares the proposed treatment with the presently accepted gold standard or placebo. There are no hard and fast rules to indicate when one passes from the second to the third phase.

One must make sure to avoid the eternal medical research pitfall of mistaking subsequence for consequence.

Types of Studies
(A) **Primary** - reports research at first hand (most common).
(B) **Secondary** - summarises and draws conclusions from primary studies

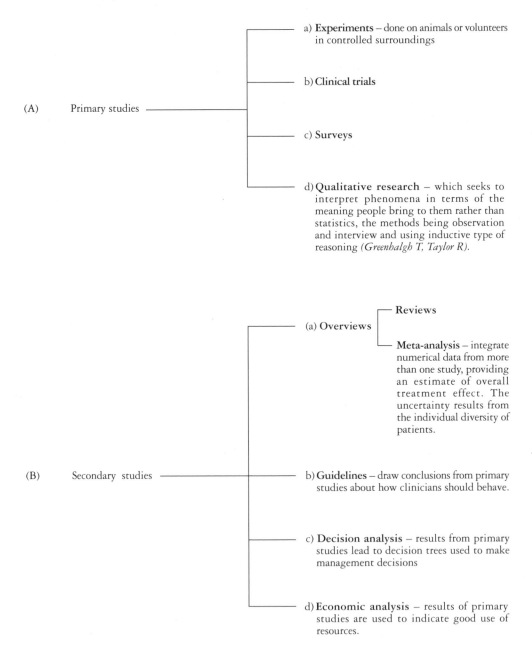

(A)   Primary studies

a) **Experiments** – done on animals or volunteers in controlled surroundings

b) **Clinical trials**

c) **Surveys**

d) **Qualitative research** – which seeks to interpret phenomena in terms of the meaning people bring to them rather than statistics, the methods being observation and interview and using inductive type of reasoning *(Greenhalgh T, Taylor R)*.

(B)   Secondary studies

(a) **Overviews**

Reviews

Meta-analysis – integrate numerical data from more than one study, providing an estimate of overall treatment effect. The uncertainty results from the individual diversity of patients.

b) **Guidelines** – draw conclusions from primary studies about how clinicians should behave.

c) **Decision analysis** – results from primary studies lead to decision trees used to make management decisions

d) **Economic analysis** – results of primary studies are used to indicate good use of resources.

Experimental Designs
The following is the most commonly used classification of designs, listed in order of hierarchy of evidence i.e. the relative weight which each type of study carries:

(a) Systematic reviews and meta-analysis
(b) Randomised controlled trials
(c) Cohort studies
(d) Tracker studies
(e) Case-control studies
(f) Surveillance studies
(g) Cross sectional surveys
(h) Case-series reports
(i) Case reports.

The latter four types of studies are sometimes grouped under the term: 'Descriptive Studies'. These deal with individuals. Ecological correlation studies deal with populations.

It is here pertinent to point out some of the jargon used in these studies:

Parallel group comparison -   Two groups entered at the same time receive different treatments and results are compared.

Paired (matched-pairs) comparison - Patients are grouped or paired according to some characteristics to balance confounding variables, receive different treatments and the results analysed in terms of differences between pairs. The fact that patients are paired does not mean they are identical and so errors may arise.

Within subject comparison - Subjects are assessed before and after an intervention and results are analysed.

Single blind -   Subjects do not know which treatment they are receiving.

Double blind -   Subjects and investigator do not know which treatment is given to whom.

Crossover -   Each subject receives both the intervention and control treatment. The principal drawback is that the effect of one treatment may carry over and affect the result of subsequent treatments. There must thus be a 'no-treatment period' between consecutive therapies.

Factorial design -   Permits investigation of the effects, separately and combined, of more than one independent variable on a given outcome. Any interaction, whether synergistic or antagonistic may be detected.

(a) **Systematic reviews, Meta-analysis and adjusted indirect comparisons** – Systematic reviews are overviews and summaries of primary studies according to a rigorous methodology which is explicit and reproducible. They are not just aids to clinical decision making, but have a much wider scope. Systematic reviews may lead to more fruitful primary studies and prevent the undertaking of unnecessary ones *(Petticrew, M.)*. Such reviews that show consistent results are more likely to provide reliable research evidence than single studies or non-systematic reviews. Meta-analysis integrates the numerical data from more than one study that ask the same research question and use identical methodology. The Achilles tendon of these studies is the fact that many trials are systematically weak and this may well be transmitted into false conclusions of systematic reviews and meta-analysis. Assessing the quality and quantity of clinical trials is obviously important. Summary scores e.g. quality scales, have been proposed for this purpose but are not recommended to identify the quality of a clinical trial *(Juni, P., Altman, D.G., Eggar, M.)*. These methods may, however, be useful for comparing different trials. One obtains better guidance by concentrating on the assessment the methodology and the potential biases of the particular trial.

When direct evidence from randomised trials is lacking or insufficient, adjusted indirect comparisons of trial results are often used. The results are usually reliable and compare well with the results of direct studies, provided that the included trials are similar and are themselves valid.

(b) **Randomised Controlled Trial Design** - The participants are randomly allocated (by lot) to either an intervention or other group. Both groups are followed up for a specified period and analysed in terms of outcomes defined at the outset. Generalised evidence needs randomised controlled trials with a corresponding variation of subjects, taking care not to exclude relevant particular categories. The work must be done independently, free from prejudice and economic constraints. Comparing a new treatment with a placebo, when a proven 'effective' treatment exists, is wasteful and unethical. It may even overestimate the effectiveness of the new therapy. In some trials randomisation may be impractical or even impossible and prospective design difficult e.g. studies testing the hypothesis of foetal origins of adult disease.

Advantages

(i) Allows rigorous evaluation of a single variable in a precisely defined patient group.

(ii) Prospective design - i.e. data are collected on events that happen after the decision for the study is taken.

(iii) Uses hypothetico-deductive reasoning which seeks to falsify rather than confirm its own hypothesis.

(iv) Potentially eradicates bias by comparing two otherwise identical groups.

(v) Allows for meta-analysis (combining its results with those of other similar trials at a later date).

Disadvantages (or Potential Deficiencies)
(i)   Time consuming and expensive.

(ii) Sample or period may be too limited.

(iii) Large institutions who fund the research project may have a vested interest and may dictate the research agenda.

(iv) Failure of randomisation.

(v) Assessors not blind to randomisation.

(vi) The ethical problem – a patient randomised to the experimental treatment may be exposed to an unknown (though 'consented') risk, while a patient randomised to a control may be deprived of the opportunity offered by the new and potentially improved treatment.

The following information is essential in the presentation of such trials:
1. The total number of patients involved in the trial.
2. Ineligible patients.
3. Eligible patients who refused consent. (The latter two points are important to assess applicability of the study.)
4. The number of patients randomised in each arm of the study.
5. The reasons for excluding patients after randomisation.
6. Indication of patients crossing over between treatments after randomisation.
7. The number of randomised patients lost to follow-up. (The balance between groups is potentially lost when patients withdraw.)
8. Assurance of adherence to the 'Uncertainty Principle'. This states that a patient is only enrolled in a randomised controlled trial, if there is substantial uncertainty (equal bet) about which of the trial arms would benefit the patient most. The fact that the researchers do not know, or strongly suspect, the result of their trial, reflects adherence to the uncertainty principle. 'Equipoise' occurs when the probability of expected outcome is equal in each arm of the trial i.e. when the uncertainty principle is maximal *(Djulbegovic, B. et al.)*.

Randomised Controlled Trials in Surgery

In contrast to the strict licensing regulations that are applied to new drugs, robust evidence and validation is often lacking for the introduction of new surgical techniques and technologies and also for many current gold standards. The application of minimally invasive techniques to a whole spectrum of purposes is one example. When challenged using scientific methods, these techniques are sometimes found to be lacking. For example, arthroscopic intervention for osteoarthritis is no better than the effect of a placebo *(Moseley, J.B., et al.)*.

Randomised controlled trials in surgical research pose special problems: Surgery is not ideally suited for placebo controlled trials because of the possibility of significant morbidity in the placebo arm, which raises obvious ethical objections. They are often underpowered, in the sense that the numbers involved cannot be as elevated as in other disciplines (a surgical procedure is more laborious and lengthy than administering a pill). Furthermore, the differences between the arms of a surgical controlled trial tend to be smaller especially when dealing with relatively rare conditions. The inherent variability and multifactorial nature of surgery poses additional problems: Operator skill, which is a very important factor for outcome, is most variable, e.g. the laparoscopic Nissen fundoplication results in Community Hospitals in the USA report a success rate of 55% which is very low compared to the > 90% reported from various specialised centres *(Peters, J.H. et al.)*, *(Cuschieri, A. et al.)*. There is a practical difficulty in carrying out research on conditions requiring emergency surgery. There is also a problem in the relationship of the timing of the surgical procedure to the operator's learning curve and in standardizing the surgical procedure itself. There is an obvious difficulty (though not an impossibility) to do double blind or single blind trials when actual surgery is performed. Blind outcome assessment e.g. of complications of surgery, is hardly possible. There is often a problem in recruitment of patients for RCT's involving surgical procedures especially because of pre-conceived preferences on the part of the patient, his relatives or his family physician. There may be a psychological resistance because of fear of the effects of the results of research on personal attitudes and interests. On top of all this, surgical research attracts funds less readily from private sectors such as the pharmaceutical industry, in part because of an admittedly poor level of research methodology in surgery in the past, but possibly also because of competition from more fashionable and glamorous fields can give this sector a more reliable financial return. This latter consideration carries a silver lining in that the consequent independence decreases the chance of bias.

On the other hand, where the role of surgery is unproven, where surgical innovation is not backed by adequate evidence, where the patient's subjective symptoms are used as outcome measures, especially if the pathology is not life threatening, then an effort should be made to evaluate surgical treatment using RCT's, especially placebo controlled trials. The role of comparative analysis still remains a most important method but one must take into account the deficiencies in evidence from the existing gold standard *(Ridgway, P.F., Darzi, A.W.)*. Recent research methodological developments many of the above mentioned difficulties in applying RCTs to surgery are surmountable *(Lilford, R. et al.)*.

One may attempt to find solutions to the above problems by:
(i)   The routine and comprehensive collection of data.
(ii) Continuous evaluation, which indicates situations where RCT's are possible.
(iii) Learning curves and variations in technique should be recognised, quantified and taken into account.

The chosen endpoints in clinical trials pose other problems: If one adopts survival as an endpoint in trials of therapy for lethal diseases e.g. cancer, this may mean that a potentially valuable therapy may be delayed for many years. One may try to avoid this problem by using other endpoints such as quantifiable clinical symptoms, quality of life data as well as biomarkers and surrogate data, provided that the clinical relevance of the latter two factors is undisputed.

   Other specialties are effected by particular difficulties in carrying out research, with obvious repercussions on evidence–based practice: In paediatrics, there may be ethical problems, such as informed consent and the protection of the child, who is the subject of the research project, from harm. There are also methodological difficulties peculiar to paediatric research, since outcome measures, which are acceptable in adults, may not be appropriate in children. Besides, the proportion of chronic diseases in children is proportionately smaller, and in addition, they are more heterogenous *(Smyth, R.L.)*. All this results in a dearth of good paediatric research with the expected effects mentioned above. In one estimate, evidence – based practice in paediatrics amounts to only 40%. The only practical suggestion to improve this situation is to make special efforts to gain the collaboration of parents, and where possible, of the children.

   Controlled trials may take the form of several subtypes;

e.g. 'Explanatory trials'- these measure the efficacy of a treatment on a homogeneous population. i.e. ideal conditions in a research clinic.

'Pragmatic trials' - measures the benefit the treatment produces in routine clinical practice, reflecting variation between patients and indicates choices between treatments *(Roland, M., Torgerion, D.)*. Pragmatic trials are helpful in cost evaluation involved in healthcare policy decisions. Their most important measure is the arithmetic mean.

When a research trial is planned or evaluated, there are two important conditions to consider: (i) The main aim should be the search for the truth of public health relevance. (ii) Patients should not be harmed by taking part in the trial.

Contining our discussion of types of experimental designs, these other types require a short description.

(c)   **Cohort Studies** - Two or more groups of people are selected or the basis of differences in exposure to a particular agent and followed up to see how many in each group have a particular outcome.
Thus cohort studies are done on patients who may or may not develop a disease, or to determine the prognosis of patients having a disease. Thus follow-up needs to be long.

(d)   **Case-control studies** - Patients with a particular disease or condition are identified and matched with controls.   Data on past exposure to a possible cause of the disease or condition are then collected.
These studies are usually concerned with aetiology. Though they are lowly placed in the hierarchy of evidence in that the link between cause and effect is not certain (post hoc, ergo propter hoc), these studies are useful to investigate rare conditions.

(e)   **Cross-sectional Surveys** - A representative sample of patients are studied to gain answers to a specific clinical question using simple methodology. Data collected at a single time but may be retrospective e.g. using case notes. These studies are very useful for estimating prevalence of a disease and are often used in public health for planning purposes..

Sample
of patients
reflective
of general
pop.

(f)   **Case Reports** - The medical history of a single patient is described. A number of these may be collected to form a case-series showing an aspect of the condition, treatment, or adverse reaction to treatment.
Descriptive studies, i.e. case reports, case-series reports, cross-sectional studies, surveillance studies and ecological correlation studies are useful in trend analysis, health care planning and hypothesis generation leading to more rigorous studies. They have inherent limitations: (i) they lack clear, specific and reproducible case definition, (ii) one may be misled into confusing "subsequence for consequence i.e. the Fallacy of the Consequent, (iii) there can be no conclusion regarding causation if there is no comparison group *(Grimes, D.A., Schulz, K.F.)*.

Q

(g)   **Qualitative Research** – This addresses questions, which cannot be tackled by experimental methods (e.g. randomised controlled trials) and clinical epidemiology. It is applied to problems involving doctors' and patients' beliefs and preferences and how clinical evidence can be applied in practical circumstances. Though the potential to obtain generalised statements from such research is conceptual rather than numerical, it may yet sensitise the clinician to issues, which he can then elaborate with his patients and thus help to bridge the gap between scientific evidence and clinical practice *(Green, J., Britten, W.)*. Qualitative research tends to answer the question 'What?' rather than 'How often?' helping us to understand the nature, strength and interactions of variables *(Black, N.)*. It may also illustrate the consumer perspective. Data are collected in non-tabular format by relatively unconstrained observation, review of archives, or by asking the subjects to respond in their own words.

(h) **Tracker trials** – These are usefully applied to rapidly changing technologies where waiting for stability may make randomisation impossible or unethical. They consist of randomised comparisons of various examples of a new type of technology with the golden standard treatment, allowing comparisons between the different treatments. Thus poorly performing treatments are detected early and are improved or rejected. When stability is reached this information is very useful. This type of trial requires more complex analysis of its findings *(Lilford, R.J.)*.

Preferred Study Design for Particular Fields of Research

This apparent abundance of designs and methods may give an impression of chaos. However one must realise that different research questions call for different types of research and designs:

(i) Therapy - Randomised Controlled Trial or a well conducted meta-analysis of several of these. A good example is The Early Breast Cancer Trialists' Collaborative Group's meta-analysis involving 55 trials on the effects of adjuvant Tamoxifen. (EBCTCG) on early breast cancer 10 year survival.

(ii) Diagnosis i.e. Testing a new diagnostic aid - Cross sectional survey of both new test and old standard. An example of this is the1994 comparison of PSA with prostatic core biopsy in the diagnosis of carcinoma of the prostate *(Catalona, W.J. et al.)*.

(iii) Screening - Cross sectional survey similar to the example given above is useful.

(iv) Prognosis - Longitudinal cohort study. A classical example is the study on the effects of smoking on British doctors by *Bradford Hill, Doll, R. and later Peto, R.*

(v) Aetiology - Cohort or case-control study depending on how rare the disease is *(Greenhalgh, T.)*. An example of the latter was the publication indicating the association of thalidomide and phocomelia *(McBride, W.G.).*

The evaluation of results of clinical research employs various mathematical and statistical procedures. It is outside the scope of this discussion to deal with this aspect except in so far as to encourage the reader to acquaint himself with basic mathematics and statistics.   *Chi-test ; Statistics; Probability.*

A number of books on this subject have been written specifically for workers in, and consumers of, clinical research. One should thus be able to view the experimental designs and methods critically. To give an example: when survival is assessed as a statistical evaluation, one must distinguish between crude survival rate and corrected survival rate (the latter takes into account the inevitable death rate in the population studied). Even corrected survival rate may not be such a good objective method of assessment because it does not take into account the quality of life.

Clinical assessment can seldom have the mathematical accuracy that a pure scientist would require. Few clinical measurements can be more than approximations. When assessing the validity of a new therapy non-experimental methods are best avoided since they so often lead to false-positive conclusions about efficacy. Reviewing several randomised trials is, without doubt, more informative. Exceptions arise in specific situations e.g. successful interventions in otherwise fatal conditions, or when the situation is pressing and there is no time for trials to be conducted. In these situations one combines the 'next best' external evidence with one's clinical expertise and proceeds within the rules of logic or probabilities, with the awareness of the dangers of coming to wrong conclusions, or correct conclusions from faulty premises.

Randomised controlled trials and observational studies are often seen as mutually exclusive methods of clinical research. This is not strictly correct though they are usually used in different settings. To date, randomised controlled trials have been considered as the gold standard, but recent literature indicates that observational studies, especially cohort and case-control studies merit more consideration. When well conducted, observational studies can quite consistently produce results similar to those of randomised controlled trials. Thus in trials evaluating the results of beta-blockers after recovery from myocardial infarction, a restricted cohort study produced essentially the same results as the Beta-blocker Heart Attack Trial, i.e. a 33% reduction in mortality over a three year period, against 28%. This is not an isolated example. This correlation also holds for other important trials including ones on the effectiveness of BCG and others exploring the relationship of screening mammography and mortality from breast cancer *(Concato, J., Shah, N., Horwitz, R.I.).*

On a theoretical basis one would avoid randomised trials if observational studies have shown marked harmful or beneficial effects, or if the postulated effects or outcomes are so small that sample size in a randomised trial would have to be prohibitively large. Randomised trials are more useful where one expects modest postulated effects and outcomes. Discarding observational evidence is a waste. On the other hand, abandoning randomised controlled trials in favour of observational studies may prove to be unscientific in most cases *(Ioannidis, J.P.A., Haidich, A.B., Lau, J.)*. One could quote several instances when the results of observational studies were subsequently convincingly disproved by subsequent RCT's: The supposed protective effect of hormone replacement therapy (HRT),on the risk of coronary artery insufficiency as indicated by epidemiological studies, was more than disproved by well-conducted RCT's *(Beral, V. et al.)*. There have been similar experiences with the results of observational studies on the effects of beta-carotene on cancer incidence and vitamin E on the incidence of myocardial ischaemia Perhaps, increasing the required significance levels for observational studies to more exacting levels, as well as more care in avoiding biases (e.g. selection and information bias) and confounding, would help avoid such conflicting and confusing information as in the examples mentioned.

There is an obvious need for more research into the relative merits and indications of the various research designs.

Deficiencies

Errors in published medical research, especially in randomised trials, are all too common. The study by Assmann S. shows the frequency of such deficiencies in work published in highly reputable journals. The CONSORT guidelines, especially the revised recommendations, *(Moher,D.)* and the QUOROM statement *(Moher, D. et al.)* are intended to help all concerned to limit these deficiencies, improving the reporting of an RTC, helping the consumer of research, as well as editors and peer reviewers to appreciate its conduct and assess the strengths and limitations of the study and the value of its results. The revised CONSORT statement includes a 22-point checklist and a flow chart applicable to RTC's and other designs. Research protocol review by journals is one of the ways journals can become involved in the primary prevention of poor quality research. This aids transparency and easy appreciation of methods and results but does not address other important facets such as readability and scientific content.

When analysing randomised controlled trials one first compares the characteristics, including prognostic factors, of the groups of patients being compared. The two groups should be, as far as possible, similar in the relevant characteristics.

The reasons for rejecting a paper may be one of the following:
1. It does not address an important scientific issue.
2. The study is not original.
3. It does not test the author's hypothesis.
4. The original protocol was compromised in the course of the study
5. The sample size was too small.
6. Inadequate control.

7. Inadequate statistical analysis.
8. Poor logic
9. Interest of authors in obtaining specific conclusions i.e. Bias of researcher.
10. Non-adherence to the 'uncertainty principle'.

Possible deficiencies in clinical research may be classified as follows:

A) **Failures of Follow-up**
    a) Absence of follow-up.
    b) Inadequate follow-up   (i)   Too short
                                                     (ii)   Failure to trace (perhaps concealed or not obvious)
                                                   (iii) Unreliable method (e.g. Postal enquiry)

    c) Inaccurate data obtained at follow-up.

B) **Failures of Definition**

    a) Vague diagnosis e.g. terms like 'peptic ulcer', 'inflammatory bowel disease', non-specific abdominal pain.
    b) Imprecise signs and symptoms e.g. weight loss, anorexia (not quantified).

C) **Failures of Assessment**

a) Faults in Experimental Techniques:
    (i)   Time difference - in the interval many other factors may have changed.
    (ii)   Poor statistical design.
    (iii)   Differing sex incidence.
    (iv)   Age difference.
    (v)   Social/Economic differences.
    (vi)   Patient selection - i.e. non-representative group.
    (vii) Policy differences in categorising patients.
    (viii) Failure of randomisation. (Selection Bias)

b) Faults in Assessment
    (i)   Inadequate statistical analysis.
    (ii)   Detection and assessment bias.
    (iii)   Poor logic e.g. Illogical conclusions, such as: Diets rich in B-carotene protect against cancer development, but this does not necessarily mean that B-carotene is the protective agent. Again, long segment Barrett's oesophagus, which is associated with oesophageal carcinoma, is assumed to be a consequence of GORD. On this basis it is held that GORD is one of the causes of oesophageal cancer. There is evidence, however,

(Gerson, L.B. et al.) that long segment Barrett's oesophagus is as common in asymptomatic individuals as in patients with GORD.

When to Stop a Trial

1. When the primary answer is clear, that is, an overwhelming evidence of superiority of the new treatment, or a not so overwhelming accumulation of evidence that it is harmful.
2. Scientific futility due to: (a) Inadequate improvement in efficiency.
   (b) External evidence from other trials giving ready answers to the questions investigated in the trial.
3. Poor research trial e.g. badly planned or performed, or else not leading to any answers *(Evans, S., Procock, S.)*.

Research Ethics Committees

The problem of harmful medical research came to the surface in the sixties *(Beecher, H.) (Pappworth, M.)*. The British scientific establishment took twenty years longer than its American counterpart to institute Ethics Committees. We observe a similar delay in setting up mechanisms for dealing efficiently with research misconduct *(Farthing, M., Horton, R., Smith, R.)*. Medical schools do not put enough emphasis in their curricula on the concepts of academic ethics and academic misconduct.

Research Ethics Committees act on behalf of the subjects of research to protect them from unnecessary risks and doubtful practices. They face several challenges: The increasing volume, type and complexity of research, failure to do research synthesis, the creation of multicentre research committee systems on top of the local bodies and the detection of scientific malpractice and fraud *(Blunt, J. et al.)*. Scientists, including medical scientists must be educated about good and bad research ethics. The need for an independent agency to guard against research fraud, plagiarism and piracy, a sort of research policeman, is tangible. This cannot be left to the editors on one end or the consumers of research on the other. The entry of false research material into the medical practice is as dangerous as any other fraud and the medical and lay consumers should be protected from this. The Office of Research Integrity in the United States and the British Research Councils in U.K. are detailed to deal with research misconduct. Maybe research ethics committees could have their terms of reference extended to include this.

It is pertinent to ask at this stage which research ethics committee is involved in 'international research collaborations', more specifically those carried out in third world countries? In such instances it is important to make sure there is a truly informed consent with clear indications of potential risks and benefits and preferably, collaboration and involvement at all stages, of the populations subjected to the research. Protecting research subjects is not only the responsibility of governments but also of those carrying out and those who consume research. The latter should make their voice heard when the necessary precautions have obviously been omitted. One could think of various measures to protect the safety of participants in clinical research. These could include the setting up of safety monitoring committees, heightened awareness by ethics and other committees that are detailed to approve research and improved communication between the various bodies. One must stress the patients' autonomy and the respect for ethical values in all who are involved in research. The implementation of informed consent, voluntary participation and confidentiality requires mutual trust between the researchers and the participants in the study. However noble the intentions, however utilitarian the goals, these should not take precedence over the freedom of will of the subjects of the research. Above all the latter should not be exploited. Furthermore, there must be clear rules where the potential conflict between the profit of industry and the needs of society, do not adversely effect the patients' best interest.

Extrapolation of this argument leads us to the present controversy on the cloning of embryo stem cells: Religious ethics has its clear norms and rules which can, and should, be expressed, but cannot be imposed on a secular state which may not have the same norms and rules. Thus religion may assume that an embryo, even in its earliest stages, is a human individual, but this may not be universally accepted by the lay or even by the scientific community. This is the essence of the present controversy. On the other hand, coining terms such as 'pre-embryo' is just an exercise in sophism, which will lead us nowhere. Stem cells need not necessarily come from human embryos, but may be obtained from reprogrammed adult cells and from placental cells. At present, 99% of embryo stem cells used in research are obtained from 'spares' from in vitro fertilization. It is possible to keep these cells in suspended animation for a period at the end of which they can take two paths: They may be allowed to die or they may be used for cloning organs or parts of these. Though one may argue that the procurement and preservation of such cells is in itself unethical, there is no doubt that such a situation exists. One has to consider which of the above-mentioned paths is the most laudable or the least despicable. This discussion does not concern the cloning of a human as a whole entity.

Reader's Assessment of the Study

It is essential to sharpen one's critical appraisal skills so as to make better use of medical research, keeping in mind the inevitable subjective element in the interpretation of data.

There are six main questions that have to be answered in assessing how worthwhile a study is:

1. Does this study add to the known literature in any way?

2. Is the study applicable to your own practice?

To answer this question one must know, who were the subjects of the study, the inclusion and exclusion criteria, and whether the study was carried out in actual clinical circumstances that you normally work in. Simplistic application of trial results, which represent an average outcome, may well have a mean positive, rather than, negative results, but may nonetheless harm some patients.

3. Was the design of the study acceptable?
   One must look deep into the type of intervention under study and the control. The reliability of the <u>units of measurement</u> used may be quite variable or impossible to estimate with confidence, let alone certainty e.g. <u>pain, anxiety</u>.

4. Bias is any systematic deviation of an observation from the true clinical state. It is a flaw in the design that leads to a built-in likelihood that the result is false. <u>Was systematic bias avoided</u> or minimised? i.e. Was there anything that induced false conclusions about groups and that distorts comparisons?

5. Was the assessment blind?   *Terminology : Single blind / Double blind .*

6. Were sample size, duration of follow-up and completeness of follow-up ascertained?
   With this notion in mind, and armed with a basic knowledge of mathematical symbols and expressions, the consumer of clinical research is in a better position to accept or reject the scientific 'information' he is exposed to.

Checklist for Reading Articles

In deciding whether a paper is worth reading it is convenient to scrutinise the different parts of the article systematically:

(a) The abstract
   (i)   Is the topic important?
   (ii)   Is the purpose of the study clearly stated?
   (iii) Is the outcome of the study clearly stated?
   (iv)   Are the results applicable to one's practice?
   (v)   Are the results statistically significant?
   (vi)   Are the results clinically significant?

(b) The introduction
   (i)   What is already known about the subject?
   (ii)   What new information does this article contribute?

(c) Method
    (i)   Is the study design appropriate?
    (ii)   Is the follow-up period long enough?
    (iii) Are the inclusion and exclusion criteria clear?
    (iv) Are the measures reliable?
    (v)   Are the statistical methods clearly outlined and reliable?
    (vi) Is the sample size and power (i.e. the number of patients needed to find the desired outcome) clearly stated?

(d) In a clinical trial
    (i)   How are subjects recruited?
    (ii)   Is there adequate randomisation?
    (iii) Is there a good control group?
    (iv) Is the study blind or double-blind?
    (v)   Is compliance evaluated?

(e) In a cohort study
    (i)   How are subjects recruited?
    (ii)   Are they randomly selected from an eligible pool?
    (iii) Is there adequate follow-up?

(f) In a case-control study
    (i)   Is subject selection random?
    (ii)   Is the control group bias-free?
    (iii) Are the records reviewed independently?

(g) In a cross-sectional study
    (i)   Are the questions unbiased?
    (ii)   Is selection random?
    (iii) What is the response rate?

(h) In a meta-analysis
    (i)   Method of collection of studies.
    (ii)   Is there clear indication on how studies are included or excluded?
    (iii) Has there been an adequate attempt to reduce publication bias?
    (iv) Is there information on how many studies are necessary to change the conclusion.

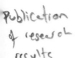
Publication of research results

(i) The results
    (i)   Do the results answer the research question?
    (ii)   Are the differences in the arms of the trial reported as actual values?
    (iii) Are there any confounding factors?
    (iv) If diagnostic procedures are being studied, is the sensitivity, specificity or

predictive value given?

(v) Are any of he studies included, systematicalle weak?

Is this researched is preliminary questions for research grant?

(j) The conclusion and discussion
- (i)   Are the research questions adequately discussed?
- (ii) Are the conclusions logical or justified?
- (iii) Are the deficiencies of the study addressed?

• Is the treatment /findings applicable ?

—→ Cost of production
—→ Mode of administration
—→ Duration of treatment

Systematic Bias

There are many types of systematic bias – Sackett has, so far, listed 56 types. Such taxonomies of bias usually indicate technical problems that can be fixed, though they are difficult to remedy once they have occurred. These are not necessarily negative as long as they are taken into account. In a way, recognition of bias helps to deepen our understanding of methodology. Imprecision, on the other hand, results from random error and this can be evaluated statistically. Precision can be improved by boosting sample size and by combining results in a meta-analysis. Researchers are duty bound to eliminate or diminish systematic bias, or alternatively, admit its presence. Different study designs call for different steps to reduce systematic bias *(Greenhalgh, T.)*. One must admit, that the idea of science as totally objective is unrealistic and does not take into consideration the human element in scientific inquiry. This subjectivity is in itself a source of several possible interpretation biases *(Kaptchuk)*. Since it is difficult to quantify the subjective elements of interpretation, one tends to sweep the problem under the carpet. Rather than ignoring this, awareness of this subjectivity renders our assessment of evidence more honest, logical and accurate.

(a) Randomised Controlled Trials

- (i)   Selection bias - Knowledge or suspicion of the treatment to be used for the next patient may effect the investigator's decision whether or not to admit the patient to the trial. One must avoid incomplete randomisation. This may happen if the randomisation is done using odd / even numbers on the ID card, date of birth, date of presentation etc.; patient or doctor chooses the treatment; or patients treated in the past are used for comparison. One example was the study showing a lower post-operative mortality following open prostatectomy when compared with that following TURP. This was explained because patients with significant comorbidity and a higher perioperative risk, were preferentially assigned to the TURP arm. Proper randomisation comes nearest to achieving control over known and unknown confounding factors.
- (ii) Performance bias - one must avoid differences in the care provided to the different groups.

(iii) Exclusion bias - differences in withdrawals from the trial. An example of this was the MRFTT randomised trial investigating risk factors in ischaemic heart disease. There was non-compliance in one limb, whilst subjects in the other limb inadvertently adopted healthier habits.

(iv) Detection bias - A new diagnostic technique detects the disease at an earlier stage giving the impression that survival is longer. To illustrate this: Statistics for lung cancer cases treated in 1953-54 had a lower 6 month survival rates for each stage of the disease than a similar group treated in 1977. In fact, newer imaging had resulted in staging of cases in the 1977 group in a more advanced stage than the would have been using 1953-4 technology resulting in differences in outcome assessment.

(v) Non-adherence to the uncertainty principle – This principle states that the fundamental criterion for eligibility to a RCT, is that both patient and doctor are uncertain about treatment appropriateness in both limbs of the trial. An illustration of this type of bias is the study comparing the post-operative hospital stay after laparoscopic cholecystectomy with minilap or open cholecystectomy. The shorter post operative stay recorded after lap chole, vanished when all staff and patients were blinded as to the type of operation. If there is already a treatment of proven value, this should be given to the patients in the control arm, e.g. the SEARCH study comparing the effects of a daily dose of 80mgs. of simvastatin with 20mgs., since the latter dose had already been shown to be beneficial. This principle may be violated when: (1) Patients are enrolled into trials with clearly inferior comparative arms, including inappropriate use of placebo comparison, or (2) Decision by the sponsor to prevent publication of negative results

(vi) Sex bias – Trials which admit a lower proportion of one sex e.g. females, than would be statistically expected, are suspect.

(vii) Financial bias – Too much emphasis in the research question concerning the interests of industry and insufficient attention given to patients' views. More specifically, basic research directed at common diseases in less developed countries should be somehow funded independently of the profit motive. Researchers and academics should make their voices heard in this respect.

(viii) Identity bias - Satellite commercial symposia during large scientific meetings help to finance the meetings. However, they often intentionally blur the distinction between what is scientific and what is commercial. This could be called the 'Faust factor', whereby the learned society sells its soul and with it truth and transparency *(Horton, R.)*.

(ix) Bias from omitted research – This occurs when, in the presence of medical topics, which are common and call out for more research to be done, yet this is not undertaken for dubious reasons. One such reason could be the improbability of good financial return from the research. Research is sometimes omitted when current practice, which is producing an excellent financial return has not been adequately investigated. The slow development of glues in surgical research may be one example of this. In other words, there would be a danger that more appropriate research would give negative results with adverse financial repercussions for the industry or category concerned. The Cockrane Collaboration is one attempt to counteract this type of bias.

(x) Ignoring regression to the mean (and other statistical errors) – Any characteristic which is different from the average tends to move towards the average after any intervention. This statistical effect is a group phenomenon and is applicable to diagnostic tests, therapy, public health, health care management and clinical audit. It occurs whenever a non-random sample is selected from a population and two imperfectly correlated variables are measured. The regression to the mean is more pronounced, the more the value of the variable is from the mean, and the less the correlation between the two variables.

(b) Non-Randomised Controlled Trial
If baseline differences between groups are great these will invalidate the conclusions.

(c) Cohort Studies
The groups studied can hardly ever be identical except for the factor that is being studied. Complex statistical adjustments have to be made to correct baseline differences. One has to be sure that these adjustments are adequate.

(d) Case-control studies
The suitability of the case studied is a determining factor.

(e) Qualitative Research
Need for quantification (ie. how often?) renders such studies inapproprate for this purpose.

To be of use to the reader, the work must be relevant, taking into account its goals. One has to query: (i) Was the study worth the effort? (ii) What were the goals? (iii) Was the design appropriate? (iv) Was the sampling fair? (v) Was the data collection and analysis sufficient and scientific? *(Mays, N. and Pope, C.)*

Interpretation (Subjective) Biases

Interpretation of data is inevitably subjective. The problem of subjective interpretation in appraisal of research has already been referred to earlier in this

Confirmation bias:	Evidence that supports one's own preconceptions is weighted differently than that which contradicts these preconceived notions. This process usually occurs unintentionally and has been demonstrated experimentally *(Kochler, J.J.)*.
Rescue bias:	This is a deliberate attempt to evade evidence that contradicts expectations. The frantic attempts to shoot down the Million Woman Study on HRT by supporters of this therapy are one example.
Auxiliary hypothesis bias:	Ad hoc modifications are introduced to imply that the findings would have been different had the experimental conditions been otherwise, thus saving a favoured hypothesis. One example is again provided by the debate on the benefits of HRT. Faced with strong evidence that HRT does not after all, benefit the incidences of ischaemic heart diseases, supporters of HRT point out that more modern forms of HRT have since become available. This could obviously become an never-ending process.
Mechanism bias:	This occurs when the underlying science provides credibility to the research findings, inducing the consumer of research to be less critical. One example was the initial reluctance to accept Helicobacter pylori as an aetiological agent for peptic ulcer because of the belief that the acid anti-bacterial barrier in the stomach was absolute.
'Time will tell' bias:	Scientific scepticism is part and parcel of the scientific process but the amount of scientific confirmation necessary before acceptance of evidence varies widely amongst scientists. At the extremes this constitutes bias and it is hard to tell what is good judgement and what is error. One example is provided by the late acceptance of proton pump inhibitors as acceptably safe treatment for peptic ulcer.
Orientation bias:	Research results seem to be affected by what the researcher is looking for, with experimental error mostly favouring the supporting hypothesis. This may be an effect of 'publication bias' or faulty design. This effect has been studied experimentally *(Rosenthal, R., Fode, K.L.)*. and is a frequent finding in the less scientific trials sponsored by the pharmaceutical industry eg trials for the validity of endotoxin antibodies in the treatment of endotoxic shock.

chapter. This can be expressed in several types of biases *(Kaptchuk, T.J.)*, which can lead to either sound judgement or errors. The result can only be judged in retrospect. All this should not lead one to a hopelessly sceptical attitude to scientific evidence, because of the subjective element in science. Accumulation of data will eventually convince. However one should always keep the human element in mind when appraising medical evidence.

Applying the Results of Research Trials and Meta-analysis

Ideally the best evidence used in clinical decision making should have a reliable and easily interpreted scientific basis. The use of 'p values', i.e. the sum of probabilities of events that might have happened but did not, and confidence intervals hardly satisfy any of these two conditions *(Shakespeare, T.P. et al.)*. The use of confidence levels, clinical significance curves and risk-benefit contours may provide easier and more reliable methods of assessment of research results, pointing out irrelevant results and underpowered studies. They should not, however, be used in isolation and their interpretation requires a well-developed inclination to statistical evaluation.

Teleoanalysis

In contrast to meta-analysis, teleoanalysis relies on combining data from different classes of evidence rather than from different studies of the same type. This synthesis of different types of evidence gives information on the quantitative relationship between the cause and the risk of a disease, and the degree of preventability of a disease.

Attitudes to Evidence

Once one is convinced of the validity of the conclusions of research one may adopt two attitudes:

(a) Lumping – a broad interpretation: The overall findings of the clinical trial or meta-analysis may be applied to individuals. This attitude makes it easier to detect bias and is therefore more reliable in indicating that evidence for a therapeutic principle is insufficient. There is also less risk of false conclusions and exploratory analysis of results. Furthermore, development of hypothesis for future research is encouraged.

(b) Splitting – a narrow interpretation: One matches the characteristics of particular patients to particular subgroups in the trials or meta-analysis. The effectiveness of a particular therapy may be confirmed, but the results are less reliable because bias is less easily detected.

Research in Developing Countries

Development funds can best help medical research in developing countries if the research is centred locally, is adapted to local needs and the beneficiaries are involved in the organisation, planning and partly in the financing of the projects. The local researchers should be able to make the necessary specific requests for funding, thus generating enthusiasm and initiative. One important requirement would be that the recipients of funds ensure efficiency and transparency, perhaps by adequate audit of the use and results of these funds.

Conclusion

Practically all scientific statements in surgery contain critical, and therefore refutable observations; their conclusions are not absolute truths but predictions proposed cautiously and with the recognition that they are transitory. These predictions or conclusions however, help to make surgical decisions. This is a humbling, if not depressing, thought which in my opinion is quite realistic. Serious research studies will, perhaps, add a point or two in favour of a hypothesis. The accumulation of such data forms the basis of meta-analysis. On the other hand education, and this includes continuing medical education, may be defined as the training that gives the ability of the conscious selves of Popper's Second World (i.e. subjective knowledge stores in the neuronal mechanisms of the brain) to grasp and understand the objective knowledge of Popper's Third World (i.e. absolute truths independent of any knowledge about them). So through continuing medical education, which is a means to an end, of which the proper consumption of clinical research is an integral part, we may come nearer and nearer to these absolute truths, but never quite reaching them, in the same way as a graph approaches its mathematical limit. On the way along this path, with continuous assessment of methods and outcome evaluation, we will get the critical conclusions which help us manage our patients, hopefully better.

Due to the inherently uncertain nature of our work, no amount or quality of research in medical or supporting sciences, can possibly lead us to the point of perfect health or eternal bliss. Our decisions and treatments may not predictably and inevitably lead to total and permanent cure, even when we follow the state-of-the-art golden rules indicated by the most laudable recent advances.

The paths ahead are not straight, some are rough and some have not been built. But by better evaluation, dissection and digestion of research on disease and the methodology of its management, we shall be in a better position to help our patients.

Chapter 7

Tailpiece

Quotation:

   Mark Twain (1835 – 1910): 'It ain't what people don't know that hurts them, it's what they know that ain't so.'

Medical theory and practice are perpetually evolving and in a state of flux. This may pose difficulties for the medical student and the practicing clinician, but it is also one of the factors that make medicine an interesting and exciting pursuit. The problem of evolution of ideas is hardly limited to medicine. Even such a basic idea as, for example, 'concepts', has undergone evolution and elaboration in the philosophical sphere:

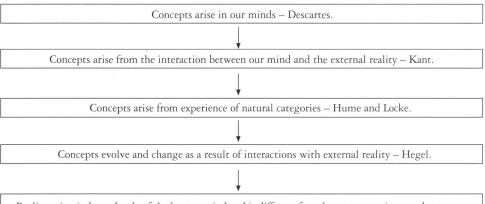

Concepts arise in our minds – Descartes.

Concepts arise from the interaction between our mind and the external reality – Kant.

Concepts arise from experience of natural categories – Hume and Locke.

Concepts evolve and change as a result of interactions with external reality – Hegel.

Reality exists independently of the human mind and is different from human experience and concepts. Ones approach is essentially a problem-solving one, replacing hypothesis with better hypothesis, rather than adding new 'certainties' to existing ones. The search for certainty has to be given up because it is not available. No general theory can be finally proved, but it can be tested and disproved. A statement that cannot be tested and possibly disproved, cannot be regarded as scientific. – Popper KM.

It is therefore understandable that the concept of disease and its management, being intrinsically relative and probabilistic, should be, even to a greater extent, subject to change, which hopefully may constitute an improvement.

The purpose of this work was to identify deficiencies in some facets of currently used surgical methodology and point out alternatives, while accepting limitations even in these. This was done in the conviction that what has been painfully developed over many years of clinical experience, can be passed down to our successors in surgery early on in their career so that the wheel of surgical progress moves forward whilst turning (even if by a factor of 2r), instead of again starting from methodological scratch. The learner is thus given a head start in his lifelong quest to help his patients.

The application of Aristotelian 'Practical Reasoning' to clinical practice is surely not original, in the sense that many doctors use such methods unconsciously. I have attempted to dissect and illustrate such goal-seeking methods so that they can be formally taught and consciously clinically applied. The intention is to be more effective, rather than just to save time, though the latter may occasionally also follow. The accumulation of data without direction, with all its consequences is thus discouraged.

Even with these methods one must accept that surgical practice is inherently uncertain and most processes are probabilistic. If both doctors and patients accept this concept, abandoning the illusion of medical certainty, then realistic decisions would become acceptable to both sides, with improvement of the doctor - patient relationship. There is always a metaphorical price to pay for any surgical decision and it is often this price, which is a source of dissatisfaction on the patient's part. Such methods require an educational system, which is able to respond to changes in the outside world by teaching scientific attitudes and thought-processes as well as scientific facts especially in key periods of medical training. The curriculum should be adapted to the changing doctor - patient relationship, promoting multi-professional teamwork and techniques of teamwork. The curriculum should also include the inter-relationship of disease and poverty, which is probably the No.1 health problem worldwide, and this training should include community field practice and community health development education. One cannot concentrate on health whilst ignoring poverty. Statistics about causes of death may be helpful but it is equally important to indicate what renders people unhealthy, miserable and hopeless.

Our efforts should be directed to make best use of current evidence in clinical decision making. Several aids in reaching this aim have been discussed in the previous chapters, which include Clinical Algorithms, Formal Decision Analysis comprising concepts of utility, probability, threshold, sensitivity analysis, and Evidence Based Medicine. The uses and limitations of these methods have been outlined. Basically they aid but do not replace clinical judgement. The clinician is faced with the pressing problem of deciding on the next step in patient management and this depends on adequate data collection and analysis leading to a working diagnosis. Thus the emphasis of further examinations and investigations will lean towards the more likely diagnosis in a way that any investigative procedure that is performed carries a potential of altering or effecting management.

It is reasonable to think that as the science factor in medicine slowly expands and replaces to a degree the less tangible 'art', results will become more accurate. This feeling is in line with the general modern belief in science and technology, especially if results are obtained in numerical, graph-form or imaging. Clinical data is often considered approximate while science and technology provide doctors with reproducibility and standardisation. Though undoubtedly valuable in patient management, one has to accept that technologies are influenced by the human hand that operates them and the human mind that evaluates the results *(Reiser, S.J.)*. One often hears that a particular diagnostic modality e.g. Ultrasound scanning is 'operator dependent'. This is surely correct, but then what isn't? Taking a medical history, setting up an intravenous infusion, making a clinical decision, performing an operation and practically everything else is equally operator dependant. Technologies, which improve accuracy, speed and dependability of data, are essential to modern surgical practice. They should, however, be used in conjunction with the clinician's own skills and not be allowed to displace the personal approach to the patient or undermine the doctor's confidence in his acumen.

The ideal clinical world would involve undeniable data, which lead to perfectly logical surgical decisions. This situation is hardly ever encountered in clinical practice since hardly ever is data pathognomonic and clinical decisions are almost always estimates of probabilities and balancing trade-offs. In this atmosphere of uncertainty, it is obvious that errors inevitably happen. One worries, however, when mistakes are too frequent or clearly avoidable. Gross and consequential errors usually happen when there are a series of small failures in different potential safeguards or rules, occurring concurrently, in sequence or in synergy. These failures may be unsafe acts by people in contact with patients, or faults within the system itself e.g. understaffing, overcrowding, poor ambient design, unreliable or non-ergonomic apparatus. The correct response to errors is to develop a defence system of safeguards, where errors are acknowledged, detected, intercepted and mitigated by proper training, testing and monitoring. This is by far more useful than blaming individuals. It also renders medical care more resilient, reliable and in a better condition to respond to difficult and adverse situations.

There is a school of thought, which regards the practice of medicine, (primarily referring to the medical practice in the U.S. but perhaps also elsewhere) as part of a wider process of industrialisation and bureaucratisation in society. The medical profession is accused of having deluded the public into believing that it has a valuable body of knowledge and skills and has created such dependence through the medicalisation of life that it has now undermined and taken away the public's right to self determination *(Illich, I.)*. Though one can see some truth in these views, especially the implications involving the interests of powerful groups and industries, it is undoubtfully hard and unjust on the honest, hardworking clinician. One has to admit that the media and medical advertising have influenced the public into regarding personal problems, ordinary ailments and risks as diseases and mild symptoms as serious (medicalisation). The process of medicalisation is neither imaginary nor static. Its effects vary in a dynamic equilibrium, some forces control these effects whilst others encourage them. The increased awareness of the public, assisted by technology, may result in a better assessment of what medicine can really offer. On the other hand some patients may obtain financial or moral benefit from having their condition categorised as a disease. Some doctors may welcome the new pastures resulting from medicalisation. The pharmaceutical and medical technology industry, have an obvious vested interest, while the media thrive in the sensationalism that this process fosters. Even politicians and the judiciary may see in it the possibility of minimalising issues and providing simplistic medical solutions for complex problems. As a result, doctors are faced with many negative aspects of life about which they can do little or nothing. The management of such problems should lie within the sphere of competence of the individual, the family or the community. Whilst increased funding of medicine is probably inevitable and also welcome, one must resist the illusion that increased resources will eventually lead to the elimination of illness, pain and death. The effect may be negative in that it may dampen our capacity to face reality. Ivan Illich pointed this out in 1974, but because of the overall optimistic atmosphere in medicine at the time, was conveniently labelled as a burnt out case. A quarter of a century later, when there is much more concern and mistrust in the various aspects of medicine, he is regarded with more respect. In this scenario doctors are set in the role of victims rather than rogues.

Though it is often assumed that decisions taken with regard to medical hazards and uncertainties are science-based, this is not exactly what happens in practice. Because of fear of contingent harm and sometimes to satisfy requests from pressure groups, the precautionary principle is often applied. Thus when a procedure, technology or drug is suspected as posing a serious or irreversible harm to human health or the environment, precautionary measures that prevent the possibility of harm, are taken even if the causal link is unproven or weak or the harm is unlikely to occur. This is an understandable attitude based on caution and precaution *(Berry, C.)*. It is also quite obvious that such inferences and actions are not highly scientific or perfectly logical. It is most unlikely that we can develop any system that will protect from harm following innovation or, indeed, any intervention.

It is important for the clinician to be aware of the stages in adoption of new technologies (vide. Innovation- Decision System - Chap 4; p 56). One should learn new technologies, but these should not be used widely until reliable evidence of their benefit becomes available. One should watch against both rigid conservatism and uncritical enthusiasm. Learning a new technique is often a painful process for clinicians that consider themselves masters of a more established one. It is not easy to learn a new technique and retain proficiency in the 'older' technique, which will be used less often as a consequence. New techniques tend to displace old skills, though these may, in time, be resuscitated and presented as new. However, since newer techniques are almost always presented as being superior, developing expertise in such methods (e.g. minimal-access surgery, trans-urethral vaporisation, laser treatment) delivers an illusion of increased professional status and is a disincentive to further what was good in earlier skills. The clinician that faces a new technological modality must find a way to understand the basic principles underlying it. This will help him evaluate whatever advantages or disadvantages it has over alternative technologies, including cost-benefit considerations. This latter consideration is only one factor in the complexity of surgical decision making.

New technologies applied in the medical sphere, will inevitably lead to the development of new disciplines and occupational groups in the delivery of health care, while some traditional ones may wither away. This will, undoubtedly, lead to tensions amongst the various occupational groups unless there is a shift of emphasis in the 'medical' education and training, as well as better organisation of integrated, interdisciplinary strategies. The scholarship of integration has not, to date been sufficiently emphasised, resulting in late clinical application of well developed strategies and technologies. This does not necessarily mean that one group takes over the responsibility of another, but rather that skills are developed to a maximum in a way that they can be complementary. This attitude should be adopted at an institutional level, which, though difficult, should not prove prohibitive, considering the common goal shared by different work groups in health care and the traditional interdependent (not inter-exchangeable) nature of their relationship.

The relationship between patients, doctors, industry, editors and owners of medical journals, administrators and politicians is affected by the relative agendas of each of these categories. The influences and pressures may be considerable, resulting in tensions, and perhaps, decisions of convenience. All these categories, medical journals included, should focus on the public's health as their primary aim and should guard against being distracted from this course by other interests, however pressing and practical they may be. There is more than a suspicion of widespread systematic bias, in medical journals, against diseases that are rife in the least developed regions of the world *(Horton, R.S.)*. As a result, published work does not honestly reflect the actual burden of disease in our planet.

Despite the degree of uncertainty that goes with the results of research, we need this scientifically generated knowledge as our data for practical reasoning and decision making on the similarly uncertain clinical situation. We are thus duty bound to continually accumulate, evaluate, discard and store the results of clinically applicable research in the most efficient way possible, though the sheer volume of such data makes this objective challenging and elusive. Continuous medical education is our lot from our student days and throughout our active life (Plate 8.). Since we do not live in an ideal world, this educational process has to be regularly evaluated to have tangible results on the profession and consequently on the patients' health. This is a small price we have to pay for the attenuation of the much greater difficulties our patients have to face. It would be foolhardy to expect such

Plate 8

C.M.E. is our lot...

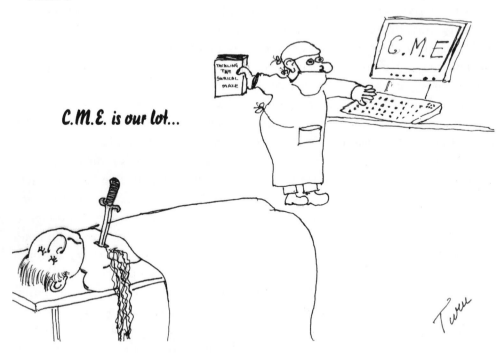

maintenance of competence to eliminate the intrinsic probabilistic nature of clinical practice. Only by clinical expertise combined with training in assessment of studies can one decide on the applicability of the results of published research. Medical training should include the teaching of efficient methods of critical evaluation of new 'external clinical evidence'.

Proper consumption of such data should bring us nearer to the absolute truths, which we can never hope to reach.

References

Adab, P., Rouse, A.M., Mohammed, M. and Marshall T. 2002.
Performance league tables: The NHS deserves better. BMJ. Vol. 324, p95-98.

Adams, D.H., Brooks, D.C. et al. 1998.
Am. J. Surgery. Vol. 155, p93.

Albanese, M.A. and Mitchell, S. 1993.
Problem-based learning: A review of literature on its outcomes and implementation issues.
Academic Medicine. Vol. 34, p52-81.

Alberti, K.G.M.M. 2001.
Medical errors: A common problem. BMJ. Vol. 322, p501-502.

Alizadeh, A.A., Eisen, M.B. et al. 2000.
Distinct types of diffuse large beta cell lymphomas identified by gene expression profiling.
Nature. Vol. 403, p503-511.

Al-Shahi, R. and Warlow, C. 2000.
Using patient-identifiable data for observational research and audit.
BMJ. Vol. 321, p1031-2.

Anbar, M. and Reisler, S.J. 1984.
Penetrating the Black Box: The Machine at the Bedside. Cambridge University Press.
Ch. 2, p23-34.

Angell, M. 2000.
Is academic medicine for sale? Editorial: New England Journal of Medicine.
p1516-1518.

Anthony, J.C. 2001.
The promise of psychiatric enviromics. British Journal of Psychiatry. Vol. 178, s8-s11.

Ascombe, G.E.M. 1978.
On practical reasoning. In: Practical Reasoning. Cornell University Press.
p33-45.

Assmann, S., Pocock, S.A., Enos, L. and Kasten, L. 2000.
Subgroup analysis and other misuses of baseline data in clinical trials.
The Lancet. Vol. 355, p1064-1069.

Badley, E.M. and Tennant, A. 1997.
Epidemiology. In: Goodwill CJ, Chamberlain MA, Evans C, eds.
Rehabilitation of physically disabled adults. 2nd ed. Stanley Thornes.

Balteskard, L. and Rinde, E. Dec. 1999.
Medical diagnosis in the internet age. The Lancet. Vol. 354, p14.

Barbour, V. and Horton R. 2002.
Mechanisms of disease. The Lancet. Vol. 358, p2.

Barton, S. 2001.
Using clinical evidence. BMJ. Vol. 322, p503-504.

Bashook, P.G. and Parboosingh, J. 1998.
Recertification and Maintenance of Competence. BMJ. Vol. 316, p545-8.

Battles, J.B. and Shea, C.E. 2001.
A system of analysing medical errors to improve GME curricula and programs.
Academic Medicine. Vol. 76, p125-133.

Bayer, 2001.
Fetzer Conference on Physician: *Patient Communication.* Academic medicine.
Vol. 76, p390-392. No.4.

Beecher, H. 1996.
Ethics and clinical research. New England Journal of Medicine.
Vol. 274, p1354-1360.

Bennett, J. 2001.
Oesopagus: Atypical chest pain and motility disorders. BMJ. Vol. 323, p791-794.

Bennett, N.L. et al. Dec 2000.
Continuing medical education: A new vision of the professional development of physicians.
Academic Medicine. Vol. 75, No12, p1167-1172.

Beral, V., Banks, F. and Reeves, G. 2002.
Evidence from randomised trials on the long term effects of hormone replacement therapy.
The Lancet. Vol. 360, p942-944.

Berger, A. 2002.
How does it work? Bone mineral density scans. BMJ. Vol. 325, p484.

Bergkvist, L., Frizell, J., Liljegren, G., Celebioglym F., Damm, S. and
Thorn M. 2001.
Multi-centre study of detection of false-negative rates in sentinel node biopsy for breast cancer.
BJS. Vol. 88, No.12, p1644-1648.

Bernard, A. 1996.
Resection of pulmonary nodules using video-assisted thoracic surgery.
Annals of Thoracic Surgery. Vol. 61, p202-204.

Berry, C. 2002.
Nonsense and non-science. Q J Med. Vol. 95, p131-132.

Berwick, D.M. 1989.
Continuous improvement as an ideal in health care. The New England Journal of Medicine.
Vol. 320, p53-56.

Berwick, D.M. 1996.
A primer on leading the improvement of systems. BMJ. Vol. 312, p619-622.

Berwick, D.M., Leape, L.L. 17.07.1999.
Reducing errors in medicine. BMJ. Vol. 319, p136-137.

Beyerstein, B.L. 2001.
Alternative Medicine and common errors in reasoning.
Academic medicine. Vol. 76, No.3, p230-237.

Burkelo, C. 1947.
Tuberculosis case findings. J.A.M.A.; Vol. 133, p354-65.

Bittner, M., Meltzer, P. and Chen, Y. 2000.
Molecular identification of cutaneous melanoma by gene expression profiling.
Nature. Vol. 406, p536-540.

Black, D.A.K. 1986.
The logic of medicine: Diagnosis. Oliver and Boyd. Ch. 3, p29-57.

Black, N. 1994.
Why we need qualitative research. Journal of Epidemiological Community Health.
Vol. 48, p425-6.

Blunt, J., Savuliscer, J. and Watson, A.J.M. 1998.
Meeting challenges facing research ethical committees. BMJ; Vol. 316, p58-61.

Borleffs, J.C.C., Custers, E.J.F.M., van Ging, J. and ten Cate O. 2003.
Clinical reasoning theatre: A new approach to clinical reasoning.
Academic Medicine. Vol. 78, p322-325.

Bosc, C. 1999.
Report to the society of neurological surgeons clinical meeting, Pasadena, California.

Boyer, E.L. 1990.
Scholarship reconsidered: Priorities of the professoriate.
The Carnegie Foundation for the advancement of teaching.

Bradbury, J. 2000.
Journey to the centre of the body. The Lancet. Vol. 356, p2074.

Brandeau, M.L. and Eddy, D.M. 1987.
The workup of the asymptomatic patient with positive faecal occult blood test.
Medical Decision Making. Vol. 7, p32-46.

Briggs, J. 1992.
Fractals: The patterns of chaos. Simon and Schuster.

Briggs, T.P., Mc Donald, D., Gardener, J.E. and Mundy, A.R. 1998.
Special Report: Prospectives. Vol. 6, No. 4, p6-8. Stirling Press Ltd.

Brugarolas, J., Haynes, B.F. and Nevins, J.R. 2001.
Towards a genomic-based diagnosis. The Lancet. Vol. 357, p249-250.

Bull, C., Yates, R., Sarkar, D., Deanfield, J. and de Leval, M. 2000.
Scientific, ethical and logistical consideration in introducing a new operation: A retrospective cohort study from paediatric cardiac surgery. BMJ. Vol. 320, p1168-1173.

Bulstrode, C. and Hunt, V. 2000.
What is mentoring? The Lancet. Vol. 356, p1788.

Burke, K. 1999.
Surgeons' College Launches Campaign To Save Research.
BMJ. Vol. 913, p1221.

Burrows, H.S. 1985.
How to design a problem-based curriculum for the pre-clinical years. Springer Verlag.

Bursztajn, H., Feinbloom, R., Hann, R. and Brodsky, A. 1990.
Medical Choices, Medical Chances. Routledge.

Bussuyt, P.M., Reitsma, J.B., Bruns, D.E. et al. 2003.
Towards complete and accurate reporting of studies of diagnostic accuracy: the STARD initiative. BMJ. Vol. 236, p41-44.

Butt, W. and Neuhausen, D. 1984.
The machine at the bedside - The machine at the marketplace.
Ch 9, p139-40. Cambridge University Press.

Campbell, E.J., Scadding, J.G. and Roberts, R.S. 1979.
The concept of disease. BMJ. 6193, p757-762.

Campbell, H., Hotchkiss, R., Bradshaw, N. and Poreous M. 1998.
Integrated care pathways. BMJ. Vol. 316, p133-36.

Canadian National Breast Screening Study. 2000
Journal of the National Cancer Institute. Vol. 92, p1490-1499.

Cannon, I.M. 1952
On the social frontier of medicine. Harvard University Press.

Card, W.I. and Good, I.J. 1978.
A logical analysis of medicine in a companion to medical studies. Ch 60. Blackwell;

Carnall, D. 2000.
Medical software's free future. BMJ. Vol. 321, p976.

Casseels, W., Schoenberg, A. and Graboys T. 1978.
Interpretation by physicians of clinical laboratory results. N Eng J Med. p299-999.

Catalona, W.J., Hudson, M.A., Scardino, P., Richie, J.P., et al. 1994.
Selection of optimal prostatic specific antigen cutoffs for early diagnosis of prostatic cancer.
Receiver operator characteristic curves. J. Urol. Vol. 152, p2037-2042.

Charatan, F. 2002.
The great American mammography debate. BMJ. Vol. 324, p432.

Clain, A. 1986
Hamilton Bailey's demonstrations of physical signs in clinical surgery. p264. Wright.

Clarke, C.Z., Hayward and O'Donnell T.F. 1990/1991.
Tutorials on surgical decision making. Theoretical Surgery. Springer Verlag International.

Coffey, R.J. et al. 1992.
An introduction to clinical paths - Quality Management in Health Care.
Vol. 1, p45-54.

COGS: Conference on Guideline Standardization. 2003.
Annals of Internal Medicine. Vol. 139, p493-498.

Collur, J. 1998.
Patient information leaflets and prescriber competence. The Lancet. Vol. 352, p1724.

Collier, J.A., Verhulst, S.J., Williams, R.G. and Norcini, J.J. 1989.
Reliability of performance on standardised patient cases: a comparison of consistency measures based on generalisability theory. Teach Learn Med. Vol. 73, p97-98.

Concato, J., Shah, N. and Horwitz, R.I. 2000.
Randomised controlled trials and the hierarchy of research designs.
New Engl. J. Med. Vol. 342, p1887-1892.

Coulter, A. 1998.
Evidence based patient information. is important, so there needs to be a national strategy to ensure it. BMJ. No. 7153, p225-26.

Cox, K. 1999.
Doctor and patient: Exploring clinical thinking. New South Wales University Press,

Crockford, M. St. Luke's Hospital, Malta.
Personal Communication. 1997.

Cunha, B.A. 2001.
Effective antibiotic-resistance control strategies. The Lancet. Vol. 357, p1307-1309.

Cuschieri, A. 1998.
The RCS Select Programme: Module 4; p15

Cuschieri, A. and Baker, P.R. 1977.
Introduction to research in medical sciences. Churchill Livingston.

Cuschieri, A. and Giles, G.R. 1982.
Essential surgical practice. Wright.

Cuschieri, A., Hunter, J., Wolfe, B., et al. 1993.
Multicenter prospective evaluation of laparoscopic antireflux surgery: preliminary report.
Surg Endosc. Vol. 7, p505-510.

Cuschieri, P. - St. Luke's Hospital Malta.
Personal communication.

Custers, E.J., Stuyt, P.M. and De Vries Robbi'. 2000.
Clinical Problem Analysis (CPA): A systematic approach to teaching complex medical problem solving. Academic Medicine. Vol. 75, No.3.

Daniels, N. 2000.
Accountability for reasonableness. BMJ. Vol.321, p1300-1.

Das, A, Ben-Menachem, T., Cooper, G.S., Chak, A., Sivak, M.V. Jnr., Gonet, J.A. and Wong, R.C.K. 2003.
Prediction of outcome in acute lower gastro intestinal haemorrhage based on an artificial neural network: internal and external validation of a predictive model.
The Lancet. Vol. 362, p1261-1266.

Dauphinee, D. and Martin, J.B. Sept. 2000.
Breaking down the walls: Thoughts on the scholarship of integration. Academic Medicine.
Vol. 25, No. 9, p881-886.

Davidoff, F. 2002.
Shame: the elephant in the room. BMJ. Vol.324, p623-624.

Davidson, D.
Essays on actions & events: Clarendon Press

Davis, D. 1998.
Global health, global learning. BMJ. Vol. 316, p385-88.

Davies, D., Evans, M., Jadad, A. et al. 2003.
The case for knowledge translation: shortening the journey from evidence to effect.
BMJ. Vol.327, p33-35.

Davies, H.T.O., Hodges, C.L. and Rundall, T.G. 2003.
Views of doctors and managers on doctor-manager relationship in the NHS.
BMJ. Vol. 326, p626-628.

Dawson, B. and Trapp, R.G. 2001.
Basic and clinical biostatistics. 3rd ed. Appleton Lange.

Day, S.C., Norcini, J.J., Webster, G.D., Vinen, E.D. and Chirico, A.M. 1988.
The effect of change in medical knowledge on examination performance at the time of certification. Proc. Annu. Conf. Res. Med. Educ: Vol. 22, p139-144.

de Dombal, F.T. 1986.
How do surgeons assimilate information? Theoretical Surgery. Vol. 1, p47-54.

de Dombal, F.T. 1993.
Surgical Decision Making. Butterworth Heinemann, p2, p28, p55.

de Dombal, F.T., Horrocks, J.C. et al., 1992.
Methods of Information. Medicine. 11, p32-37.

de Dombal, F.T. 1991.
Diagnosis of acute abdominal pain. 2nd Edition. Churchill Livingston. p81-83 and 110-111.

de Dombal, F.T. 1982.
The OMGE acute abdominal pain survey. Progress report.

de Dombal, F.T. and Scand, J. 1984.
Gastroenterol. Suppl. 95. Vol. 19, p28-40.

de Dombal, F.T., Leaper, D.J. and Harrocks J.C. 1974.
Human and computer-aided diagnosis of abdominal pain. Further report with emphasis on performance of clinicians. BMJ. Vol.1, p376-380.

de Dombal, F.T., Leaper, D.J., Staniland JR, et al. 1972.
Computer aided diagnosis of acute abdominal pain. BMJ. Vol.2, p9-13.

de Ville, de Goyet, C. 2000.
Stop propagating disaster myths. The Lancet. Vol. 356. p762-64.

Delamothe, T., Smith, R., Keller, M.A. and Witscher B.
Netprints: The next phase in the evaluation of biomedical publishing.
BMJ. Vol. 319, p1515-6, 1999.

Delamothe, T. 2000.
Quality of websites: Kitemarking the west wind. BMJ. Vol.321, p843-844.

de Koning, H.L. 2000.
Assessment of Nationwide Cancer Screening Programmes. The Lancet. Vol. 355, p80-81.

De Lucas. 1734.
Essay on Waters

De Mello, E. and Sousa, C. 1994.
Camb.Q. Health Ethics. p358-366.

Department of Health, (Eng). 1989.
Working for patients. Working paper 6, Command 555. London: HMSO.

Deregowski, J.B. 1974.
Illusion and culture. In: Gregory, R.L, Gombrich, E.H. (eds): Illusion in nature and art. Scribner.

Dixon, J. and Preker, A. 1999.
Learning from the NHS BMJ. Vol.319, p1449-1450.

Dobson, R. 2001.
Limiting operations to high volume teams has wide implications. BMJ. Vol.322, p1384.

Dobson, R. 2002.
We are definitely not amused. BMJ. Vol.325, p919.

Donaldson, L.J. and Muir Gray, J.A.
Clinical governance: A quality duty for health organisations.
Quality in health care, 7 (sip): S37-S44.

Doll, R., Peto, R., Wheatly, K., Gray, R. and Sutherland, I. 1994.
Mortality in relation to smoking: 40 years observation on male British doctors.
BMJ. Vol. 309, p901-911.

Dowie, R. and Langman, M. 1999.
Staffing of hospitals: Future needs, future provisions. BMJ. Vol. 319, p1193-1195.

Drew, P.J., Cule, N., Gough, M., Heer, K., Monson, J.R.T., Lee, P.W.R., Kerin, M.J. and Duthie, G.S. 1999.
Optimal education techniques for basic surgical trainees: Lessons from education theory.
J.R. Coll. Surg. Edinb. Vol. 44, p55-56.

Djulbecovic, B., Lacevic, M., Cantor, A., Fields, K.K., Bennett, C.L., Adams, J.R., Kuderer, N.M. and Lyman, G.H. 2000.
The uncertainty principle and industry sponsored research.
The Lancet. Vol. 356, p635-638.

Eaton, W.W. and Henderson, A.S. 1995.
Looking to the future in psychiatric epidemiology. Epidemiologic Reviews.
Vol. 17, p240-242.

EBCTCG. 1998.
Tamoxifen for early breast cancer: An overview of the randomised trials.
The Lancet. Vol. 351, p1451.

Eccles, J.C. 1970.
Facing Reality. Heidelberg Scientific Library. Longman/Springer Verlag

Edelstein, R.A., Reid, H.M., Usatine, R. and Wilkes, M.S. 2000.
A comparative study of measures to evaluate medical students' performance.
Academic Medicine. Vol. 75, No. 8.

Editorial. 2001.
The Lancet. Vol. 357, p489.

Editorial. 2001.
The Lancet. Vol. 357, p817.

Editorial. 2004.
The Lancet. Vol. 363, p1247.

Egan, G. 1990.
The skilled helper. 5th ed. Constable.

Egan, T.D. and Wong, K.C. 1992.
Perioperative smoking cessation and anaesthesia: A review. Journal of Clinical Anaesthesia. Vol. 4, p63-72.

Elstein, A.S. 1991.
On the psychology of clinical intuition. Theoretical Surgery. Springer Verlag. Vol. 6, p95-97.

Elstein, A.S. Oct. 2000.
Clinical problem solving and decision psychology: Comment on 'The epistemology of clinical reasoning'. Academic Medicine. Vol. 75. No. 10, p S134-136.

Elstein, A.S. and Scwarz, A. 2002.
Clinical problem solving and diagnostic decision making: Selective review of the cognitive literature. BMJ. Vol. 324, p729-732.

Elwyn, G., Edwards, A., Eccles, M. and Rovner, D. 2001.
Decision analysis in patient care. The Lancet. Vol. 358, p571-574.

Engelberg, J. 1992.
Complex medical case histories as portals to medical practice and integrative, scientific thought. Am. Physiol, J. 263. (Adv. Physiol. Ed. 8.) S45-S54.

Enthoven, A.C. 1985.
Reflections on the management of the NHS Nuffield Provincial Hospital Trust.

Enthoven, A.C. 1999.
In Pursuit of Improving the NHS Nuffield Trust.

Eva, K.V. and Brooks, L. 2000.
The under-weighting of implicitly generated diagnosis. Academic Medicine. Vol. 75. No. 10, p S81-83.

Evans, J., Golcare, M.J. and Lambert, T.W. 2000.
Views of UK medical graduates about flexible and part time working in medicine: A qualitative study. Med. Educ. Vol. 34, p355-362.

Evans, S. and Procock, S. 2001.
Societal responsibilities of clinical trial sponsors. BMJ. Vol. 322, p569-570.

Farthing, M., Horton, R. and Smith, R. 2000.
UK's failure to act on research misconduct. The Lancet. Vol. 356, p2030.

Fayers, P.M. and Sprangers, M.A.G. 2002.
Understanding self-rated health. The Lancet. Vol. 359, p187-189.

Felice, A.G. 2002.
Of mind over ...... matter. Malta Medical Journal. Vol.15, p41-44.

Felice, A.G., Cuschieri P., Caruana Montalto, P., Cacciottolo, J. and
Zarb Adami, J. 1986.
Antibiotic policy: Government health services.

Fitts, A.M. and Posner, M.I. 1967.
Human performance. Brooks-Cole.

Frankel, S., Smith, G.D., Donovan, J. and Neal, D. 2003.
Screening for prostate cancer. The Lancet. Vol. 361, p1122-1127.

Freemantle, N. and Hill, S. 2002.
Medicalisation, limits of medicine, or never enough money to go round.
BMJ. Vol. 324, p864-865.

Freidson, E. 1970.
Profession of medicine. A study of the sociology of knowledge. Harper Collins.

Gage, F.H., Eriksson, P.S., Perfileira, E., Bjork-Erikson, T., Alborn, A.M.,
Nordberg, C. and Peterson, D.A. 1998.
Neurogenesis in the adult human hippocampus. Nat Med. Vol. 4, p1313-17.

Gallagher et al. 2001.
Ninth annual medicine meets virtual reality conference, Newport Beach, CA.

Gardner M. 2003.
Why clinical information standards matter. BMJ. Vol. 326, p1101-1102.

Garrison, F.H. 1933.
Persian medicine and medicine in Persia: A geometric survey. Bull Hist Med. Vol.1, p144.

Garvey, C.J. and Hanlon, R. 2002.
Computerised tomography in clinical practice. BMJ. Vol. 324, p1077-1080.

Gerson, L.B., Shetler, K. and Triadafilopoulos, G. 2002.
Prevalence of Barrett's oesophagus in asymptomatic individuals. Gastroenterology,
Vol.123, p461-467.

Ginzberg, E. 1990.
The medical triangle. Harvard University Press.

Girgenza, G. and Todd, P. 1999.
Simple heuristics that make us smart. New York University Press.

Global forum for health research.
The 10/90 report on health research 2000. Geneva, WHO 2000.

Godlee, F., Horton, R. and Smith, R. 2000.
Global information flow. The Lancet. Vol. 356, p1129-1130.

Goel, V. for Crossroads 99 Group. 2001.
Appraising organised screening programmes for testing for genetic susceptibility for cancer.
BMJ. Vol. 322, p1174-1178.

Gonsalkorale, W.M., Miller, V., Afzal, A., Whorewell, P.J. 2003.
Gut. Vol.52, p1623-1629.

Gorbach, S.L., Mensa, J., Gatell, J.M. 1999.
Pocket book of antimicrobial therapy and prevention. Preface. Williams and Wilkins.

Gorman, P.J., Meier, A.H., Rawn, C. and Krummel, T.M. 2000.
The future of medical education is no longer blood and guts, it is bits and bytes.
American Journal of Surgery. No.5, p353-355.

Gotzsche, P.C. 2000.
Why we need a broad perspective meta-analysis. BMJ. Vol. 321, p585-6.

Gotzsche, P.C. and Olsen, O. 2000.
Is screening for breast cancer by mammography justifiable?
The Lancet. Vol. 355, p129-133.

Graber, M., Gordon, R. and Franklin, N. 2002.
Reducing diagnostic error in medicine. What's the goal? Academic Medicine.
Vol. 77, p981-992.

GRADE. 2004.
Working group grading the quality of evidence and strength of recommendations – Norway.
BMJ. Vol. 328, p1490-1494.

Green, J. and Britten, W. 1998.
Qualitative research and EBM. BMJ. Vol. 316, p1230-32.

Greenberg, D.S. 2003.
Conference deplores corporate influence on academic science.
The Lancet. Vol. 362, p302-303.

Greenhalgh, T. 1997.
Education and Debate: How to read a paper: Getting your bearings etc.
BMJ. Vol. 315, p243-246, 422-425, 480-483, 540543, 596-599, 672-675.

Greenhalgh, T. and Taylor, A. 1997
Assessing methodological quality of published papers. BMJ. Vol. 315, p740.

Gregory, R.L. 1966.
Eye and brain: The psychology of seeing. Weidenfield and Nicholson.

Griffiths, V.G. 1994.
The medical aspects of personal injury assessment: Maltese Medical Journal.
Vol. VI, p31-35.

Grimes, D.A. and Schulz, K.F. 2002.
Descriptive studies: What they can and cannot do. The Lancet. Vol. 359, p145-149.

Grimshaw, J.M. and Russell, I.T. 1993.
The effect of clinical guidelines on medical practice: A systematic review of rigorous evaluations.
The Lancet. Vol. 342, p1317-1322.

Grol, R., Dalhuijsen, J., Thomas, S. et al. 1998.
Attributes of clinical guidelines that influence the use of guidelines in general practice: Observational study. BMJ. Vol. 317, p858-861.

Gross, R. and Lorenz, W. 1990.
Intuition in surgery as a strategy for surgical decision making. Theoretical Surgery. Vol. 5, p54-59; Springer Verlag

Gunning, K.E.J. 2001.
Scoring systems for intensive care. Surgery. Vol. 19:1, p12-14. Medicine Publishing Co.

Gyatt, G., Meade, M., Jaschke, R., Cook, D. and Haynes B. 2000.
Practitioners of evidence-based care. BMJ. Vol. 320, p954-955.

Habermann, E. 1991.
Intuition – a two-edged sword. Theoretical Surgery. Vol. 6, p85-86.

Hadorn, D.C. and Holme,s A.C. 1997.
The New Zealand Priority Criteria Report. BMJ, Vol. 314, p135-8.

Hall, J.C. 2000.
Learning to operate. Vol. 18:7, p i-ii.

Halm, F.A. and Chassin, M.R. 2001.
Why hospital death rates vary? Editorial. New England Medical Journal. Vol. 354, No. 9, p392-394.

Hamdorf, J.M. and Hall, J.C. 2000.
Acquiring surgical skills. BJS. Vol. 87, p28-37.

Hanning, I. and Dow, E. 1998.
Tumour Markers. Surgery. Medicine Publishing Company. Vol. 16:9, p iii-vi.

Harre, R. 1984.
The Philosophies of science: Science and society. Oxford University Press. Ch 7, p185-86.

Hart, E.A. 1998.
Antibiotic resistance: an increasing problem? BMJ. Vol. 316, p1255-56.

Hajdu, S.I. and Melamed, M.R. 1984.
Limitations of aspiration cytology in the diagnosis of primary neoplasm. Acta Ctol. Vol. 28, p337-345.

Heisenberg, W. 1971.
Physics and beyond. Harper and Row.

Henry Garland, L. 1960.
The problem of observer error. Bull N.Y. Academic Medicine. Vol. 36.

Hmelo, C.E. 1998.
Cognitive consequences of problem-based learning for early development of medical expertise.
Teach Learn Medicine. Vol. 10, p92-100.

Hobsley, M. 1982.
Pathways in surgical management. Edward Arnold.

Hobsley, M. 1986.
The nature of clinical acumen theoretical surgery. Springer Verlag. Ch 1, p10-18.

Hobsley, M. 1991.
Reasoning like greased lightening? Theoretical Surgery. Vol. 6 , p76-77.

Holtzman, N.A. and Marteau, T.M. 2000.
Sounding board: Will genetics revolutionize medicine?
The New England Journal of Medicine. Vol. 343, No. 2, p141-144.

Horton, R. 1999.
The uses of error. The Lancet. Vol. 353, p429.

Horton, R. 2000.
The less acceptable face of bias. The Lancet. Vol. 356, p959-960.

Horton, RS. 2003.
Medical journals: Evidence of bias against the diseases of poverty.
The Lancet. Vol. 361, p712-713.

Illich, I. 1976.
Limits of medicine - medical nemesis: The expropriation of health. Pengiun.

Ioannidis, J.P.A., Haidich, A.B. and Lau, J. 2001.
Any casualties in the clash of randomised and observational evidence.
BMJ. Vol. 322, p879-880.

Jahn, H., Mathiesen, F.K., Neckelmann, K., Hovendal, C.P., Bellstrom, T. and Gottrup, F. 1997.
Comparison of clinical judgment and diagnostic ultrasonography in the diagnosis of acute appendicitis: Experience with a score-aided diagnosis. Eur J Surg. Vol. 163, p433-443.

James, E.A. et al. 1984.
The machine at the bedside - Prospects and dilemmas of the consultant. Section D, Ch 13. Cambridge University Press.

Jones, P.F. 1987.
Emergency abdominal surgery. 2nd Ed. Blackwell Scientific Publications.

Jones, P.F., Krukowski, Z.H. and Youngson, G.G. 1998.
Emergency abdominal surgery. 3rd Ed. Chapman and Hall. p47, p51.

Jones, R. 2000.
Self care. BMJ. Vol. 320. p596.

Jones, R., Higgs, R., de Angelis, C. and Prideaux, D. 2001.
The changing face of medical curricula. The Lancet. Vol. 357, p699-703.

Jones, R.M., Rosen, M. and Seymour, L. 1987.
Smoking and anaesthesia. Anaesthesia.Vol. 42, p1-2.

Juni, P., Altman, D.G. and Eggar, M. 2001.
Assessing the quality of controlled clinical trials. BMJ. Vol. 323, p42-46.

Kamolz, T., Bammer, T. and Pointner, R. 2000.
Predictability of dysphagia after laparoscopic Nissen fundoplicaton
Am. J. of Gastroenterology. Vol. 95 (2), p408-414.

Kaptchuk, T.J. 2003.
Effect of interpretative bias on research evidence. BMJ. Vol. 326, p1453-1455.

Kausitz, J., Pecen, L.
Determination of the most applicable tumour markers for individual tumour localizations. http://www.lfp.cuni.cz/journals/bioenv/1977/1/21-en.html

Keefer, C.S. 1966.
Summary of symposium on the future of medicine. Mc Graw Hill.

Kleinert, S. 2000.
Next phase of priority-setting in health care. The Lancet. Vol. 356, p1869-1870.

Knottnerus, J.A., van Weel C. and Muris J.W.M. 2002.
Evaluation of diagnostic procedures. BMJ. Vol. 324, p477-480.

Koehler, J.J. 1993.
The influence of prior beliefs on scientific judgements of evidence quality. Organ Behav Hum. *Decision Processes.* Vol. 56, p28-55.

Koran, L.M. 1975.
The reliability of clinical methods, data and judgements.
N Eng J Med. Vol. 293, p642-46

Kostoff, R. 2001.
The extraction of useful information from biomedical literature.
Academic Medicine. Vol.76. No.12, p1265-1270.

Kranse, R., Beemsterboer, P., Rietbergen, J. et al. 1999.
Predictors for biopsy outcome in the European randomised study of screening for prostate cancer (Rotterdam region). Prostate. Vol. 39, p316-322.

Kripski, W.C. 1991.
The peripheral vascular consequences of smoking. Annals of Vascular Surgery.
Vol. 5, p291-304.

Kyle, J. 1992.
Pye's Surgical Handicraft. Duties of the house surgeon. Butterworth Heinemann. p3-5.

Larkin, M. 2000.
Clinicians need practice in 'Informed Decision Making'. The Lancet. Vol. 355, p47.

Larkin, M. 10.02.2001.
Evidence based prescribing made simple. The Lancet. Vol. 357, p448.

Le Fanu J. 1999.
The rise and fall of modern medicine. Little, Brown.

Lavelle, S.M. and Kavanagh J.M. 1995.
Clinical presentation of jaundice in Europe — occurrence and diagnostic value of clinical findigs. Euricterus project.

Law, M.R. and Wald, N.J. 2002.
Risk factor thresholds: Their existence under scrutiny. BMJ. Vol. 324, p1573.

Lazare, A. 1987.
Shame and humiliation in the clinical encounter. Archives of Internal Medicine.
Vol.147, p1653-1656.

Leinster, S.J.
SELECT: General Principles. Module 2. p13.

Lichtenstein, P., Holm, N.V., Verkasalo, P.K., Iliadou, A., Kaprio,
J., Kosinvuo, M., Pukkala, E., Skytthe, A., Hemminki. 2000.
Environmental and hereditary factors in the causation of cancer.
The New England Journal of Medicine. Vol. 343, No. 2, p78-85.

Lilford, R.J., Braunholts D.A., Greenhalgh, R. and Edwards, S.J.L. 2000.
Trials and fast changing technologies: The case for tracker studies.
BMJ. Vol. 321, p43-46.

Lilford, R., Braunholtz, J., Harris, J. and Gill T. 2004.
Trials in surgery. BJS. Vol. 91, p6-16.

Lindahl, S. Dec. 2000.
The Lancet: Perspectives. Vol. 356, p54.

Lindblom, A. and Liljegren. 12.02.2000.
Tumour markers in malignancy. BMJ. Vol. 320, p424-427.

Little, J.M. 1993.
The problem of the clinical process - A Popperian analysis. theoretical surgery,
Vol. 8, No. 3, p146-150.

Loefler, I.J.P. 1999.
The drawbacks of overspecialisation. J.R. Coll. Surg. Edin., Feb 44, p11-12.

Loff, B. and Gruskin, S. 2000.
Getting serious about right to health. The Lancet. Vol. 356, p1435.

Loong, T.W. 2003.
Understanding sensitivity and specificity with the right side of the brain.
BMJ. Vol. 327, p716-719.

Lotz, J.P. and Peters, W. 1999.
Scandinavian Breast Cancer Group: American Society of Clinical Oncology Meeting.

Lou-Yao, G., Albertsen, P.C., Stanford, J.L., Stukel, T.A., Walker-Corkery, E.S. and Barry, M.J. 2002.
Natural experiment examining impact of aggressive screening and treatment on prostate cancer mortality in two fixed cohorts from Seattle area and Connecticut.
BMJ. Vol. 325, p740-743.

Mackenzy, J. 1920.
Symptoms and their interpretation. Shaw and Sons.

Madden, A.
Research or audit? Network 1, p1.

Mallia, P.
Rights of the patient. Public lecture, University of Malta.

Mahadevia, P.J., Fleisher, L.A., Frick, K.D. et al. 2003.
Lung cancer screening with helical computer tomography in older adult smoker: A decision and cost-effectiveness analysis. JAMA Vol. 289, p313-322.

Marcus, P. et al. 2000.
J. Natl. Cancer Institute Vol. 92, p1308-16.

Martin, R.F. and Rossi, R.L. 1997.
The acute abdomen: An overview and algorithm. Surgical Clinics of North America. Vol. 77, p1227-43.

Martin, R.M., Sterne, J.A.C., Gunnell, D., Ebrahim, S., Smith, G.D. and Frankel, S. 2003.
NHS Waiting lists and evidence of national or local failure: Analysis of health service data.
BMJ. Vol. 326, p188-192.

Martling, A.L., Holm, T., Rutquist, L.F., Moran, B.J., Heald, R.J. and Cedermark, B. 2000.
Effect of a surgical training programme on outcome of rectal cancer in the county of Stockholm.
Stockholm Colorectal Cancer Group. Basingstoke Bowel Cancer Research Project. The Lancet. Vol. 356, p93-96.

Matsumoto, E.D. and Reznick, R.K. 2001.
Assessment of surgical competency in trainees. Surgery. Medicine Publishing Company Ltd. Leading article.

Mauron, A. 2001.
Is the genome the secular equivalent of the soul? Essays. Vol. 291. No.5505, p831-832.

Mayor, S. 2003.
Hormone treatment increases the breast cancer risk, study shows. BMJ. Vol. 327, p359.

Mayou, R. and Farmer, A. 2002.
Functional and somatic symptoms and syndromes. BMJ. Vol. 325, p265-268.

Mays, N. and Pope, C. 2000.
Assessing quality in qualitative research. BMJ. Vol. 320, p50-52.

Mc Adam, W.A.F., Brock, B., Armitage, T. et al. 1990.
Annals of the Royal College of Surgeons of England. Vol. 72, p140.

Mc Bride, E.D. 1948.
Disability evaluation: Principles of treatment of compensable injuries. 5th ed. J.B. Lippincott. American Medical Association.

McBride, W.G. 1961.
Thalidomide and congenital abnormalities. The Lancet. ii. p1358.

McGregor, M., Hanley, J.A., Boivin, J.F., et al. 1998.
Screening for prostate cancer: Estimating the magnitude of overdetection. Canadian Medical Association Journal. Vol. 159, p1368-1372.

McGuaran, A. 2002.
Royal College issues new guidelines on gifts from drug companies. BMJ. Vol. 325, p511.

Mc Manus, J.F.A. 1963.
Fundamental ideas in medicine. Thomas Books.

MEDMARX. 2001.
Summary of information submitted to MEDMARX in the year 2001: A human factor approach to medication errors. http://www.usp.org/medmarx

Mellor, N.E. and Horton R.G. 1995.
Art in medical forum. Medical Education Services Ltd.

Meltzer, M.I. 2001.
Introduction of health economics for physicians. The Lancet. Vol. 358, p993-998.

Miller, A.B., To T., Baines, C.J., Wall, C. 2002.
Mammography and mortality from carcinoma of the breast. Annals of Internal Medicine. Vol. 137, p305-312.

Miller, J. and Petrie, J. 2000.
Development of practice guidelines. The Lancet. Vol. 355, p82-83.

Mitton, S. 2001.
Light brought to a standstill. The Lancet. Vol. 357, p496.

Moher, D. 1998.
CONSORT: *An evolving tool to help improve quality of reports of randomised controlled trials.* JAMA. Vol. 279, p1489-1491.

Moher, D., Cook, D.J., Eastwood, S. et al. 1999.
Improving the quality of reports of meta-analysis of randomised controlled trials: The QUOROM statement. The Lancet. Vol. 354, p1896-1900.

Moher, D., Schulz, K.F., Altman, D.G. for the CONSORT Group. 2001.
The CONSORT statement: *Revised recommendations for improving the quality of reports of parallel-group randomised trials.* The Lancet. Vol. 357, p1191-1194.

Moran Campbell, E.J. 1976.
Basic science, science and medical education. The Lancet. p134-38;

Moseley, J.B., O'Malley, K., Petersen, N.J. et al. 2002.
A controlled trial of arthroscopic surgery for osteoarthritis of the knee. N. Engl. J Med. Vol.347, p81-88.

Mowatt, G., Bower, D., Brebner, J., Cavins, J., Grant, A.M., Mc Kee, L.
Health technology assessment. p149.

Moynihan, B. July 2000.
Quotation on cover. Archives of Surgery.

Murdoch, M., Kressin, N., Fortier, L., Giuffre, P.A., Oswald, L. 2001.
Evaluating the psychometric properties of a scale to measure medical students' career-related values. Academic Medicine. Vol. 76, No. 2, p157-165.

Murray, M. 2000.
Access to care. BMJ. Vol. 320, p1594-1596.

Murray, W.J.G. 1998.
Nurses in surgery – opportunity or threat? A personal view. J. R. Coll. Surg. Edinb.
Vol. 43, p372-373.

Neidhiser, J.M. 2001.
Understanding the role of genome and environment: Methods in genetic epidemiology. British
Journal of Psychiatry. Vol. 178, s12-s17.

Nel, M.R. and Morgan, M. 1996.
Pre-operative cessation of smoking. Anaesthesia. Vol.51, p309-311.

Nelson, E. 2004.
Whole body magnetic resonance imaging. BMJ Vol. 328, p1387-1388.

Neville, A.J., Reiter, H.I., Eva, K.W., Norman, G.R. Oct. 2000.
Critical appraisal turkey shoot: Linking critical appraisal to clinical decision making.
Academic Medicine. Vol. 75, No. 10, p S87-89.

Newcomb, P. et al. 2003.
Long-term efficacy of sigmoidoscopy in the reduction of colorectal cancer incidence.
Journal of National Cancer Institute. Vol. 95, p622-625.

Norman, G.R. 2000.
The epistemology of clinical reasoning: Perspectives from philosophy, psychology and neuroscience.
Academic Medicine. Vol. 10, p S127-133.

Norman, G.R. 1988.
Problem-solving skills, solving problems and problem-based learning.
Med. Educ. Vol. 22, p279-286.

Norman, G.R. and Schmidt, H.G. 2000.
Effectiveness of problem-based curricula: theory, practice and paper darts.
UK Med. Educ. Vol. 34, p721-728.

Nossal, C.J.V. 1975.
Medical science and human goals. Edward Arnold.

O'Doherty, M.J. and Marsden, P.K. 2000.
Being equipped for clinical PET. The Lancet. Vol. 356, p1701-1703.

Oneson, R.H., Minke, J.A., Silverber, S.G. 1989.
Intraoperative pathologic consultation: An audit of 1000 recent consecutive cases.
Am. J. Surg Pathol. Vol. 13, p237-243.

Otto, S.J., Francheboud, J., Looman, C.W.N., Broeders, M.J.M., Boer, R., Hendricks,
J., Verbeek, A., de Koning, H.J. et al. 2003.
*Initiation of population-based mammography screening in Dutch municipalities and effect on
breast cancer mortality: A systematic review.* Lancet Vol. 361, p1411-1417.

Oumeish, Y.O. 2000.
Scientific research, development and the human dimension. BMJ. Middle East.
Vol. 7, p6-13.

Pappworth, M.H. 1967.
Human guinea pigs: Experimentation on man. Routledge and Kegan Paul.

Parboosingh, J. 1996.
Learning portfolios. Journal Cont. Educ. Health Professions. Vol. 16, p75-81.

Parkes, C., Wald, N.J., Murphy, P. et al. 1995.
*Prospective observational study to assess the value of prostatic specific antigen as screening test
for prostate cancer.* BMJ. Vol. 311, p340-343.

Patel, V.G. and Groen, G. 1986.
Knowledge-based solution strategies in medical reasoning. Cogn. Sci. Vol. 10, p95-100.

Paton, H.J.
Translation of: Kant E. *The moral law.* p84-85.

Paulson, E.K., Kalady, M.F. and Pappas, T.N. 2003.
Suspected appendicitis. New England Journal of Medicine. Vol. 348:3, p236-241.

Perou, C.M., Serlie, T., Eisen, M.B. et al. 2000.
Molecular portraits of human breast tumours. Nature. Vol. 406, p747-752.

Peters, J.H., DeMeester, T.R., Crookes, P. et al. 1998.
*The treatment of gastroesophageal reflux disease with laparoscopic Nissen fundoplication: Prospective
evaluation of 100 patients with 'typical' symptoms.* Ann. Surg. Vol. 228, p40-50.

Petrie, K.J. and Wessely, S. 2002.
Modern worries, new technology and medicine. BMJ. Vol. 324, p690-691.

Petry, J. 2000.
Surgery. Vol. 127 No. 4, p363-368.

Petticrew, M. 2001.
Systematic reviews from astronomy to zoology: Myths and misconceptions
BMJ. Vol. 322, p98-101.

Philli,p H., Fleet, Z. and Bowman, K. January 2003.
The European Working Time Directive – interim report and guidance from the Royal
College of Surgeons of England Working Party. London. The Royal College of
Surgeons of England.

Poloniecki, J., Valencia, O. and Littlejohns P. 1998.
Cumulative risk adjusted mortality chart for detecting changes in death rate.
BMJ. Vol. 316, p1697-700.

Popper, K.R. 1962.
The logic of scientific discovery. Hutchinson.

Popper, K.R. 1989.
Conjectures and refutations: The growth of scientific knowledge. Routledge.

Pule, C.
Personal Communication.

Raffle, A.E., Alden, B., Quinn, M., Blabb, P.J. and Brett, M.T. 2003.
*Outcomes of screening to prevent cancer: Analysis of cumulative incidence of cervical abnormality
and modelling of cases and deaths prevented.* BMJ. Vol. 326, p901-904.

Ragnor Norrby, S. 1984.
Pharmacological aspects on the use of antibiotics in surgery. National Board of Health
Welfare - Drug information Committee. Sweden.

Ramor, K.D., Schafer, S. and Tracz, S.M. 2003.
Validation of the Fresno test of competence in evidence based medicine.
BMJ. Vol. 326, p319-321.

Raphs, D.N.L., Brian, A.J.L., Grimdy, D.J. and Hobsley, M. 1980.
How accurately can direct and indirect inguinal herniae be distinguished.
Br Med J. Vol. 280, p1039-40.

Rasmussen, J. and Lind, M. 1982.
A model of human decision making in complex systems and its use for design of system control strategies. Riso National Laboratory Report. Riso – M. 2349, Roskilde, Denmark.

Rawlins, M. 1999.
In pursuit of quality. The National Institute for Clinical Excellence.
The Lancet. Vol. 353, p1079-1082.

Rawlings, M.D. 2001.
Letters: *The failings of NICE.* BMJ. Vol. 322, p389.

Reason, J. 2000.
Human error: Modes and management. BMJ Vol. 320, p768-770.

Rees J. 2000.
Patients and intellectual property: A salvation for patient-oriented research.
The Lancet. Vol. 356, p849-850.

Reiser, S.J. 1981.
Medicine and the reign of technology. Cambridge University Press.

Rhodes, R.S. and Rhodes, P. 1998.
Cost-effectiveness analysis in surgery. Surgery. Vol. 123, No. 2, p119-120.

Richards, T. 1998.
Disease management in Europe. BMJ. Vol. 31, p426-427.

Ridgway, P.F. and Darzi, A.W. 2002.
Placebos and standardising new surgical techniques. BMJ. Vol. 325, p560.

Riolo V. 1995.
Introduction to logic. Philosophical studies series. 3.1-3.3. Malta University Publishers Ltd. Also: Personal communication.

Rodgers, A., Walker, N., McKee, H. et al. 2000.
Reduction of post operative morbidity and mortality with epidural or spinal anaesthesia: Results from an overview of randomised trials. BMJ. Vol. 321, p493-497.

Rodgers, E.M. and Shoemaker, F.F. 1971.
Communication of innovations. Free Press. p99-133.

Romano, P.S. and Mark, D. 1992.
Patient and hospital characteristics related to in-patient mortality after lung cancer resection.
Chest. Vol. 101, p1332-1337.

Roland, M. and Torgerson, D.J. 1998.
Understanding controlled trials. BMJ. Vol. 316, p285.

Rosai, J. 1996.
Ackerman's surgical pathology. Mosby. 8th ed. Vol. 1, p7.

Rosen, M.P., Sands, D.Z., Morris, J., Drake, W. and Davis, R.B. 2000.
Does a physician's ability to accurately suspect the likelihood of pulmonary embolism increase with training? Academic Medicine. Vol. 75, No.12, p1199-1205.

Rosenthal, R. and Fode, K.L. 1963.
Three experiments in experimenter bias. Psychol Rep Monog. Vol. 3, p12-18.

Russel, W.M.S. and Burch, R.L. 1959.
The principles of humane experimental technique. Methuen.

Rutz, W., Von Knoving, I. and Walender, J. 1989.
Frequency of suicide in Gotland. Acta Psychiatrica Scandinavica. Vol. 80, p151-154.

Sackett, D.L. and Haynes, R.B. 2002.
The architecture of diagnostic research. BMJ. Vol, p539-541.

Sackett, D.L., Rosenberg, W.M., Muir Grey, J.A., Brian Haynes, R. and
Scott Richardson, W. 1996.
Evidence Based Medicine: What is and what isn't: BMJ. Vol. 312, p71-72.

Sackett, D.L., Scott Richardson, W., Rosenberg, W.M., Brian Haynes, R. 1997.
Evidence Based Medicine. Churchill Livingston.

Satava, R.M. and Jones S.B. 1996.
Virtual reality environments in medicine: computer-based exams for board certification.
American Board of Specialities. p121-131.

Scott Butterworth, J. and Reppert, EH. 1960.
Auscultatory acumen in the general medical population. JAMA. Vol. 174, p32-34.

Schon, D.A. 1984.
Educating the reflective practitioner:Toward a new design for teaching and learning in the professions. Jossey-Bass.

Schulkin, J. 2000.
Decision sciences and Evidence-Based Medicine – Two intellectual movements to support clinical decision-making. Academic Medicine. Vol. 75, No. 8, p816-7.

Seglen, P.O. 1997.
Why the impact factor should not be used for evaluating research.
BMJ. Vol. 314, p498-502.

Sehmahl, F.W. and Weizsacker, C.F. 1998.
Medicine and modern physics. The Lancet. Vol. 351, p1291-1292.

Sen, A. 2002.
Health: Perception versus observation. BMJ. Vol. 324, p860-861.

Senior, K. 2001.
Tying the genetic sequence to human disease. The Lancet. Vol. 357, p532.

Shakespear, T.P., Gebski, V.J., Veness, M.J. and Simes J. 2001.
Improving interpretation of clinical studies by use of confidence levels, clinical significance curves and risk-benefit contours. The Lancet. Vol. 357, p1349-1353.

Shaneyfelt, T. 2001.
Building bridges to quality. JAMA. Vol. 286, p2600-2601.

Shekelle, P., Eccles, M.P., Grimshaw, J.M. and Woolf, S.H. 2001.
When should clinical guidelines be updated? BMJ. Vol. 323, p155-157.

Sheldon, A., Gayatt, G.H. and Haines A. 1998.
When to act on evidence. BMJ. Vol. 314, p139-142.

Siebers, R. and Holt, S. 2000.
The accuracy of references in five leading medical journal.
The Lancet. Vol. 356, Correspondence, p1445.

Skolnick, E.T. et al. 1998.
Anaestesiology. Vol. 88, p1114.

Slotnick, K.D. 1999.
How doctors learn: Physicians' self directed learning episodes.
Acad. Med. Vol. 74, p1106-1117.

Smith, R. 1999.
The case for structuring the discussion of scientific papers. BMJ. Vol. 318, p1224.

Smith, R. 2001.
Measuring the social impact of research. BMJ. Vol. 323, p528.

Smith, R. 2001.
Electronic publishing in science. BMJ. Vol. 322, p627-629.

Smits, P.B.A., Verbeek, J.H.A.M. and de Buisonje, C.D. 2002.
Problem based learning in continuing medical education: A review of controlled evaluation studies. BMJ. Vol. 324, p153-155.

Smyth, R.L. 2001.
Research with children. BMJ. Vol. 322, p1377-1378.

Song, F., Altman, D.G., Glenny, A.M. and Deeks, J.J. 2003.
Validity of indirect comparison estimating efficacy of competing interventions: Empirical evidence fom published meta-analysis. BMJ. Vol. 326, p472-475.

Spelcher, S.J. 2003.
Managing Barrett's Oesophagus. BMJ. Vol. 326, p892-893.

Stephenson, A., Higgs, R., Sugarman, J. 2001.
Teaching professional development in medical schools. The Lancet. Vol. 357, p867-870.

Stewart, M. 2001.
Towards a global definition of patient centred care. BMJ. Vol. 322, p444-445.

Stumpf, S.E.
Elements of philosophy: An introduction

Swales, J.D. 2000.
Science and healthcare: An uneasy partnership. The Lancet. Vol. 355, p1637-1640.

Sweetland, H.M. and Moneypenny, I.J. 1993.
Cancer screening with special reference to breast cancer. The Medicine Group.
Vol. 21, p337-340.

Swensen, S.J. 2003.
Screening for cancer with computerised tomography. BMJ. Vol. 326, p984-985.

Synnot, A. 1993.
The body social. Routledge.

Taber, L., Yen, M.F., Vitak, B., Chen, H.T., Smith, R.A. and Duffy, S.W. 2003.
Mammography service screening and mortality and mortality in breast cancer
patients: 20 year follow-up, before and after introduction of screening.
The Lancet. Vol. 361, p1405-1410.

Taylor, I. 1999.
Recent advances in surgical oncology. 4th Malta Med. School Conf.

Taylor, I. 2000.
Surgical trainees face particular problems. BMJ. Vol. 321, p301.

Technical Education Council. 1982.
Troubleshooting Charts.

The Million Women Study Collaborators. 2003.
Breast cancer and hormone replacement therapy in The Million Women Study.
The Lancet. Vol. 362, p419-427.

The Scottish Office, Department of Health. 1999.
The introduction of managed clinical networks within the NHS in Scotland. Leeds.
NHS Executive.

Tonks, A. 1999.
Registering clinical trials. BMJ. Vol. 319, p1565-1566.

Tonks, A. 2002.
The authors of guidelines have strong links with drug industry. BMJ. Vol. 324, p383.

Towle, A. 1998.
Changes in health care and continuing medical education for the 21st Century.
BMJ. Vol. 316. p301-304.

Tuddenham, W.J. 1963.
Problems of perception in chest roentgenology. Rad Elm North Am. Vol. 1, p277-289.

Tuffs, A. 2004.
Only 6 % of drug advertising material is supported by evidence. Bmj.com. news roundup. Commenting on Arznei Telegramm 2004: 35: 21-3. BMJ. Vol. 328, p485

Tutton, P. 1997.
The selection interview. J. Higher Education Pol. Manag. Vol. 19, p27-33.

U.S. Government Printing Office - Washington D.C.
Development of Medical Technology

U-205 Course Team. 1995.
Medical knowledge: Doubt and certainty. Open University Press Philadelphia. Health and Disease 2nd level.

Van den Hurk, M.M., Wolfhagen, I.H., Dolmars, D.H. and Van der Vleuten, C.P. 1999.
The impact of student-generated learning issues on individual study time and academic achievement. Medical Education. Vol. 33, p808-814.

Van der Meulen, J. 2001.
Statistical methods to compare surgical performance: Confidence intervals. Surgery. Vol. 19, p259-264. The Medicine Publishing Co. Ltd.

Van Weel, C. 2001.
Examination of context medicine. The Lancet. Vol. 357, p733.

Veitch, J. 1937.
The meditations and selections from the principles of Rene Descartes. La Salle, I11. Open Court Publishing Company.

Velanovich, V. 1994.
Reductionism in biology and medicine: The implications of fractional and chaos theory. Theoretical Surgery. Springer Verlag. Vol. 9, p104-107.

Vincent, C., Neale, G. and Woloshyniwych, M. 2001.
Adverse events in a Bristol hospital: A preliminary retrospective record review. BMJ. Vol. 322, p517-519.

Violato, C., Lockyer, J. and Fidler, H. 2003.
Multisource feedback: A method for assessment of surgical practice.
BMJ. Vol. 326, p546-548.

Von Wright. 1978.
On so-called practical inference. Practical reasoning. Oxford University Press.
p46-61.

Wade, D.T, de Jong, B.A. 2000.
Recent advances in rehabilitation. BMJ. Vol. 320, p1385-1388.

Wagner, J.M., McKinney, W.P. and Carpenter, J.L. 1996.
Does this patient have appendicitis? JAMA. Vol. 276, p1589-1594.

Walshe, K. 2002.
The rise of regulation in the NHS. BMJ. Vol. 324, p967-970.

Ward, J.P.T, Gordon, J., Field, M.J. and Lehmann, H.P. 2001.
Communication and information technology in medical education.
The Lancet. Vol. 357, p792-795.

Warner, M.A., Offord, K.P., Warner, M.E., Lennar, R.L., Conover, M.A. and
Jansson-Schumaker, U. 1989.
*Role of pre-operative cessation of smoking and other factors in post-operative pulmonary
complications: A blinded prospective study of coronary artery bypass patients.*
Mayo Clinic Proceedings. Vol. 64, p609-616.

Wass, V., Van der Vleuten, C., Shatzer, J. and Jones, R. 2001.
Assessment of clinical competence. The Lancet. Vol. 357, p945-948.

Weiner, D.A., Ryan, T.J., Mc Cabe, C.H. et al. 1979.
*Exercise stress testing correlations among history of angina, ST-segment response,
and prevalence of coronary artery disease in the coronary artery surgery study
(CASS)* N. Engl. J. Med. Vol. 301, p230-235.

Weinstein, M.C. and Fineberg, H.V. 1980.
Clinical decision analysis. Saunders.

Weiss, K.B., Mendosa, G., Schall, M.W., Berwick, D.B. and Roessner, J. 1997.
Breakthrough series guide: Improving asthma care in children and adults.
Boston Institute for Healthcare Improvement.

Weitzel, J.N. and McCahill, L.E. 2001.
The power of genetics to target surgical prevention. The New England Journal of Medicine.
Vol. 344, No. 25, p1942-4.

West, M.A. 2002.
How can good performance amongst doctors be maintained? BMJ. Vol. 325, p669-670.

Wilcox, M.H. and Warren, N.F. 2001.
Molecular diagnostic techniques. Medicine. Vol. 29, p27-30.

Williams, O. 1996.
What is clinical audit? Annals of the Royal College of Surgeons of England.
Vol. 78, p406-411.

Williams, S.J. and Colnan, M. 1996.
Modern medicine. UCL Press Ltd.

Wilmer, A. and Rutgeerts, P. 1996.
Push endoscope: Technique, depth and yield of insertion.
Gastrointest Endosc. Clin. North Am. Vol. 6, p759.

Wilson, A. 1994.
Changing practices in primary care. Health Education Authority.

Wilson, J.M. 1968.
Principles and practice of screening for diseases. Geneva: WHO.

Wilson, R.M., Runciman, W.B., Gibber, R.W., Harrison, B.T.,
Newby, L., Hamilton, J.D. 1995.
The quality in Australian health care study. Med J Australia. Vol. 163, p458-71.

Wittgenstein, L. 1953.
Philosophical investigations. Blackwell.

Wolpaw, D.R. 1996.
Early detection of lung cancer. Cancer screening and diagnosis. Vol. 80, p63-82.

Woolf, S.H., Crol, R., Hutchinson, A., Eccles, M. and Grinshaw, J. 1999.
Potential benefits, limitations and harm of clinical guidelines.
BMJ. Vol. 318, p527-530.

Wooton, R. 2001.
Telemedicine. BMJ. Vol. 323, p557-560.

World Bank. 1993.
World Development Report 1993: *Investing in health.* Oxford University Press.

World Medical Assocition Declaration of Helsinki.
http://www. wma.net/e/policy/17-c_e.html

Wright, P., Jansen C. and Wyatt J.C. 1998.
How to limit clinical errors in interpretation of data.
The Lancet. Vol. 352, p1539-1543.

Wulff, H.R. 1986.
Theoretical Surgery. Vol. 1, p18-20. Springer Verlag.

Wulff, H.R. 1981.
Rational diagnosis and treatment. 2nd ed. Blackwell.

Wyatt, J.C and Keen, J. 2001.
The new NHS information technology strategy. BMJ. Vol. 322, p1378-1379.

Yasumura, M., Mori, Y., Takagi, H. et al. 2003.
BJS. Vol. 90, p460-465.

Young, M.J., Williams S.V. and Einesberg. 1984.
The Machine at the bedside: The technological strategist: Employing techniques of clinical decision making. Ch. 10, p172-173. Cambridge University Press.

Zimmerman, R., Emery, J. and Richards. T. 2001.
Putting genetics in perspective. BMJ. Vol. 322, p1005-1006.

Index